ADVANCED DENTAL HISTOLOGY

A DENTAL PRACTITIONER HANDBOOK
SERIES EDITED BY DONALD D. DERRICK, D.D.S. L.D.S. R.C.S.

ADVANCED DENTAL HISTOLOGY

J. W. OSBORN
Ph.D., B.D.S.(Lond.), F.D.S. R.C.S.(Eng.)
Professor of Anatomy in relation to Dentistry
Guy's Hospital Medical School, London

and

A. R. TEN CATE
BSc., Ph.D., B.D.S. (Lond.)
Professor and Chairman, Division of Biological Sciences,
Faculty of Dentistry, University of Toronto, Canada

THIRD EDITION

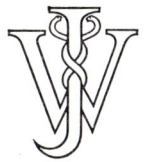

BRISTOL : JOHN WRIGHT & SONS LTD
1976

First Edition, 1967
Second Edition, 1971
Third Edition, 1976
Reprinted, 1977

ISBN 0 7236 0429 0

PRINTED IN GREAT BRITAIN BY HENRY LING LTD., A SUBSIDIARY OF
JOHN WRIGHT & SONS LTD., AT THE DORSET PRESS, DORCHESTER

PREFACE TO THIRD EDITION

NEARLY every chapter in this new edition has been revised by the addition of new material and the deletion of passages which now appear to be incorrect or out of date. About half the diagrams have been redrawn and several new diagrams have been added.

We wish to emphasize that this small book was originally, and still is, intended for undergraduates although we think that it may often be of value to postgraduates. To those who find it irritating that authors are not referred to except in the bibliographies at the end of each chapter, we would point out that this is the normal practice in undergraduate texts. Sources can usually be recognized by studying the titles of the works quoted in the bibliographies.

PREFACE TO THE FIRST EDITION

THIS book is not intended to be an orthodox textbook of dental histology but rather a supplement dealing with the latest, and often most controversial, aspects of the subject. Nor is it claimed that this book is fully comprehensive.

The rapid advances made in recent years in the field of dental histology involve the application of new disciplines, the results of which are to be found in an ever increasing range of scientific periodicals. In consequence, it has become increasingly difficult for students to find the time, and indeed the facilities, to collate this information from perusal of the original literature. Furthermore, the time lapse between completion of a manuscript and the appearance of a book is such as to preclude the incorporation of the latest information on any subject. It seemed to the authors, therefore, a worth while service to review these latest advances, and to present them in a series of short essays in the least dogmatic manner. They are based upon the dental histology portion of the pre-clinical course given to students of dentistry at Guy's Hospital. Many of the ideas presented herein are still in the formative stage and may or may not come to fruition in the future. Nevertheless, they are included in the hope of providing a stimulus for further study and enquiry on the part of the reader.

If the rapid advances in this subject over the past few years continue in the future, it is anticipated that this book will require frequent revision if it is to be of continuing value. Realizing this, the book has been written so as to facilitate rapid revision by virtue of its simplified line diagrams and absence of photographic plates.

Every effort has been made to produce an authoritative book at low cost, consistent with the policy of constant revision. Rather than burden the reader with a long list of references to each chapter, only those which are readily available in most libraries are quoted, from which further specific references can be obtained.

February, 1967

W.A.G.
J.W.O.
A.R.T.C.

CONTENTS

CHAPTER 1

THE INVESTIGATION OF TISSUES

THE aim of this chapter is to give an outline of the more important methods which are used to determine the structure and function of the dental tissues and to indicate a few of their limitations.

By far the most common tool used in the investigation of tissues is the light microscope, which in general requires the preparation of sections thin enough to transmit light. The preparation of thin sections of dental tissues necessitates either demineralization of hard tissues with the loss of the highly mineralized enamel or, if demineralization is to be avoided, the grinding of slices of dental tissue with the consequent loss of the soft tissue elements.

A wide variety of chemicals has been used to stain demineralized sections in order to make the thin, and therefore largely transparent, material visible under the light microscope. It is obvious that these stained sections appeared very different prior to being pickled (fixed), dehydrated, and wax-embedded, and yet most of our knowledge of the histological structure of the body, and much of our knowledge of how the body functions, has been learned by studying these stained remnants of the original tissue. The confidence with which interpretations are made is based on what is known as the 'reproducible artefact'.

It is of little value to mix together a number of chemicals and after staining a section with them to describe the appearance of the tissue in that one section. The proportions and concentrations of the materials and the time of staining must be carefully measured and controlled. The effect of using different proportions, concentrations, and staining times is studied and finally the combination which produces the best staining of tissue is selected. This type of experimenting is fundamental to light microscopy and many of the well-known staining procedures are named after the persons who originally formulated them (e.g., Mallory, van Gieson, Masson).

If a new tissue is to be studied, one or more of the well-known staining procedures is selected on the basis of the components of the tissues which are selectively stained by the method. The effects of the staining procedure are studied on a large number of sections until it is verified that the stain will always produce the same picture; in other words that the 'artefact is reproducible'.

Frequently we are interested in the overall appearance of a tissue rather than the minutiae of a single component contained within

1

the tissue. One of the standard combinations of stains used for general histology is that of haematoxylin and eosin. Mature haematoxylin is a basic stain and therefore attaches to acidic materials (e.g. the DNA and RNA of cells). Therefore nuclei are stained blue and cells rapidly synthesizing material (cells with a high proportion of RNA in the cytoplasm) will have a blueish cytoplasm. Eosin has an affinity for most materials and will stain all components red. It is therefore referred to as a 'counterstain'. Without this counterstain the material not stained by haematoxylin would be colourless and largely invisible.

For a more detailed study of some of the components of a tissue more selective staining procedures are required. Indeed, the value of a stain frequently depends on the specificity with which it will react with a component of a tissue. For example, certain silver solutions will precipitate on collagen, reticulin, and the axons of nerves. The brown and black artefacts produced by these precipitates may be reproducible but the value of sections stained in this way is often limited because of the difficulty in distinguishing which component of the tissue has been affected. Therefore, in the use of silver stains elaborate methods have been introduced in attempts to confine the precipitate to one specific component of the tissue.

Some of the most specific of staining techniques are those used in histochemistry. Histochemical techniques attempt to demonstrate microscopically the chemistry of cells and tissues. Such techniques usually depend on specific chemical reactions which form a coloured reaction product visible with the light microscope. An example illustrating the principles of histochemical practice is the simultaneous coupling azo-dye method for demonstrating the location of the enzyme acid phosphatase in tissue sections. The term 'acid phosphatase' is applied to the organic catalyst which, operating at an acid pH, splits phosphates from organic esters. Sections must be prepared without inactivating the enzyme or dislocating it from its intracellular position. In the case of the dental tissues this normally implies the cutting of unfixed, undemineralized frozen sections in order not to denature the enzyme. To such sections a solution is applied which is buffered at an acid pH (the working pH of the enzyme) and contains a substrate (sodium α-naphthyl phosphate) which the enzyme can split, together with a relatively colourless azo-dye. The enzyme splits the phosphate from the substrate exposing the naphthyl group which instantly combines with the azo-dye to produce a coloured reaction product at the site of the enzyme activity (*Fig. 1*). Using this method it is possible to demonstrate the activity of acid phosphatase in a wide variety of tissues.

It is sometimes helpful to view sections unstained. This is particularly true of the ground sections so commonly used in the study of dental tissues. In this case the picture seen under the microscope is produced due to differences between the light absorption, refractive indices, and optical interference of the component tissues. For instance, the dentinal tubules in a ground section are seen due to the difference of refractive index between the air contained in the tubule and that of the intertubular dentine. If the tubule becomes filled with calcified material, the tubule then has a similar refractive index to the intertubular material and the dentine becomes transparent. Probably the borders of enamel prisms are seen under the light microscope because of light reflection at the border separating adjacent prisms. The striae of Retzius appear brown by transmitted light because in the region of the striae blue light (shorter wavelength) is scattered away from the direction of viewing.

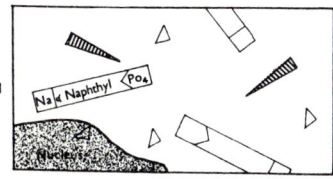

Diagrammatic appearance of section containing enzymes (cross-hatched) and nucleus (stippled). The section has been treated with sodium α naphthyl phosphate and azo-dye (triangle) in a buffered medium.

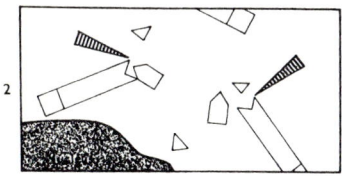

The enzyme splits off the PO_4 and the sodium α naphthyl component competes for the azo-dye.

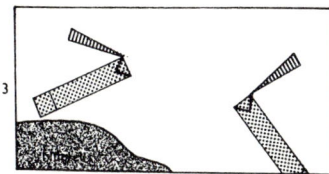

The PO_4 is replaced by the azo-dye to produce a coloured reaction product at the sites of enzyme activity.

Fig. 1.—Diagrams of the steps in the simultaneous coupling azo-dye method for demonstrating the location of the enzyme acid phosphatase in tissue section.

Frequently the optical heterogeneity of a specimen is difficult or impossible to see using the normal optical system of the light microscope. Phase contrast, interference, and polarization microscopy techniques use different optical systems to make these heterogeneities visible. For example, the phase contrast microscope will pick up very small, otherwise invisible, changes in refractive index.

3

Electron Microscopy

The limit of resolution of the light microscope (the ability to distinguish two points as separate) is dependent upon the wavelength of light. Attempts have been made to improve resolution by utilizing radiations of shorter wavelength, such as X-rays, but the difficulty here is the inability to focus X-rays; hence at present X-ray microscopy is not a practical proposition. Far greater success has been achieved, however, by the use of electron beams which, although not part of the electro-magnetic spectrum, can be produced with a much shorter wavelength than light radiation. Also, as electrons are electrically charged, they can readily be focused by means of electro-magnets. The principles of electron microscopy are the same as for light microscopy (*Fig. 2*), except that electrons are used instead of light for illumination of the specimen and electro-magnets are substituted for the glass lenses of the light microscope. Because of the short wavelength, the resolving power of the electron microscope is over 100 times greater than that of the light microscope and

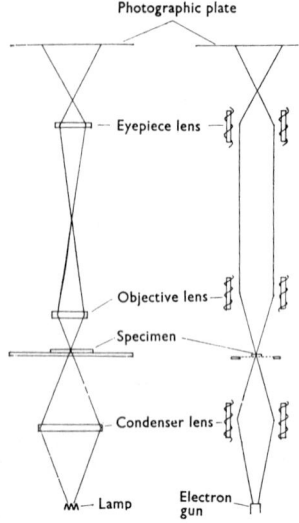

Fig. 2.—Diagram illustrating the similar principles of light and electron microscopy.

true magnifications of up to × 1 000 000 are possible. The preparation of any tissues for electron microscopy is complicated by the fact that extremely thin sections are necessary as electrons have little penetrative power, and this raises additional technical problems so far as the dental hard tissues are concerned.

Because the wavelengths of electron beams are outside the visible spectrum a black and white image of the tissue being examined is

4

produced on a screen. Many cell organelles are bounded by lipids. These can be stained with the heavy metal in osmium tetroxide which absorbs electrons. On such electron micrographs the membranes will appear dark (they have absorbed electrons).

While the electron microscope has many advantages over the light microscope, the preparation and study of sections is very much more difficult. Therefore, whereas the cells studied by the light microscopist may be numbered in thousands, only a few may be studied at any one time by the electron microscopist. This poor sampling rate limits the value of electron microscopy. Furthermore, for many years much of electron microscopy was merely descriptive. For instance, numerous types of vesicle have been described—coated vesicles, granular vesicles, dense vesicles, light vesicles, dark vesicles, and so on without much knowledge of the function of the vesicles described. It is only recently that sufficient knowledge of cell function has been acquired to enable functions to be allotted to many of the structures seen in electron micrographs of cells. Recently, histochemical and autoradiographic (*see below*) techniques have been used in electron microscopy. Such techniques have made it possible to interpret the function of some of the less obvious organelles seen by electron microscopists.

Both light and electron microscopes produce an image in two dimensions of what is substantially a two-dimensional slice of tissue. It is often difficult to visualize the appearance of the tissue in three dimensions.

In the scanning electron microscope a narrow beam of electrons is made to scan the surface of specially prepared tissues, rather like the spot on a television screen. The scanning beam is reflected from the surface of the tissue and ultimately on to a viewing screen. Because the beam obeys the normal laws of reflection an apparently three-dimensional image is produced of the surface scanned, based on the equivalent of light and shade. The image produced may be magnified up to 20 000 times.

Apart from the fact that scanning electron microscopy does not require the very demanding techniques of section cutting necessary for transmission electron microscopy (a surface is 'scanned' by electrons rather than electrons being transmitted through an ultra-thin section), the instrument has the advantage of providing an incredible depth of focus. With the light microscope at a magnification of about $\times 1\,000$ (its limit of useful magnification) less than a 1 μm depth of a section is in focus; if we want to examine the whole thickness of a 5 μm thick section we must rack the microscope up and down. But at the relatively enormous magnifications used in scanning electron microscopy, most of the irregularities of a surface being examined are in sharp focus. It is for this reason that the scanning electron microscope has been so valuable in studying, for example, the surfaces of cells and the surfaces of teeth.

Autoradiography is a more subtle form of identifying specific constituents in cells or tissues. In this instance, a substance used in normal metabolism (for instance calcium ions, an amino-acid, or a nucleic acid) is made radioactive and introduced into the living animal where it is utilized in an identical manner to its normal non-radioactive counterpart. Subsequently, this material can be traced in tissue sections due to its radioactivity. For instance, radio-active proline can be injected into the peritoneum of a rat. This proline is absorbed, circulates in the bloodstream, and becomes utilized in the formation of collagen in the periodontal ligament.

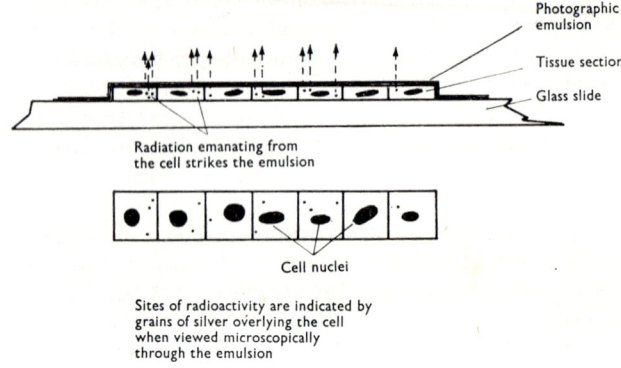

Fig. 3.—Diagram illustrating the principle of autoradiography.

At a later date the animal is killed and sections of the periodontal ligament are prepared by normal histological methods. The sections are mounted on a slide and, in a dark room, are coated with a thin layer of photographic emulsion. After a few weeks in the dark room (the actual time depends on the half-life of the labelled atom) the emulsion is reduced over the spots where the radioactive proline is present. The emulsion is then developed photographically and the section stained with haematoxylin and eosin. When the stained section is viewed through the now transparent emulsion, the silver grains indicate the exact spots where the radioactive proline has been incorporated (*Fig. 3*).

In one experiment the apices of continually growing rodent incisors were blocked with a filling material. Labelled calcium was now injected into the abdomens and a few weeks later the animals were killed. Ground sections of the incisors were cut and covered with photographic emulsion in a dark room. Subsequently it was observed that radioactive calcium had been incorporated in the newly formed enamel. Because the pulp cavity had previously been blocked, it is evident that the calcium must have come from the ameloblasts via the bloodstream proving that the enamel organ and not the pulp provided the mineral for enamel.

The above methods can all give information on structure, and the newest electron microscopes may be able to resolve atoms. But the identification of composition at the level of atoms and molecules can only be undertaken by chemical techniques.

Every protein has three levels of structure which can be analysed: the proportion of the amino-acids it contains, the order of these amino-acids in the protein chain, and lastly the three-dimensional arrangement of the resulting chain or chains. Of these levels of structure the first (the proportion of the amino-acids) is the most easy to study while the second and third are extremely difficult and not often attempted.

It is not difficult to break the peptide bonds in a protein chain, thereby reducing the protein to its constituent amino-acids. In order to analyse the proportion of these amino-acids chromatographic techniques are used. Several methods exist but the principle involved is the same. A mixture of substances is made to move through a network or filter which differentially retards those substances that have, for example, a higher molecular weight or a positive charge. For instance, in column chromatography the sample to be analysed is washed through a long column of resinous material. The resinous material may be chosen preferentially to retard positively charged amino-acids and also have a pore size which will slow down the rate of movement of all the larger amino-acids. The amino-acids pass through the column at different rates (according to their size and charge) and can be collected separately at the bottom of the column (*Fig. 4*). Subsequently the proportions of each amino-acid can be determined. The data is usually given as numbers of amino-acids per 1 000 residues. For instance, collagen in human dentine has 319 glycine molecules in every 1 000 amino-acids, i.e. the collagen contains about one-third glycine.

Microradiographic Methods: X-rays have a common application in the study of dental tissues. Most readers will be familiar with the conventional radiographs used in diagnostic medicine. Such radiographs rely on the use of X-rays generated at high voltage and of short wavelength, the so-called 'hard' X-rays. The same principle is involved with contact microradiography. The specimen is placed in contact with a recording photographic emulsion and exposed to 'soft' X-rays, generated at low voltages and of longer wavelengths. The X-rays are differentially absorbed by the specimen, depending on the number, the kind of atoms, and their capacity to absorb X-rays. From the resulting photographic record information can

7

be gained about the overall pattern, degree, and detail of mineralization. For instance, peritubular dentine can easily be recognized using microradiography.

Experimental Methods: Such methods usually depend upon altering the environment of the living tissue being studied in a specific way and observing any response with many of the techniques already described. Included in this category are experimental methods such as those designed to reveal the effect of specific dietary deficiencies and additions, ablation studies, and tissue culture studies. There are many other techniques in this category which have been used to investigate the dental tissues. Examples will be referred to in later chapters.

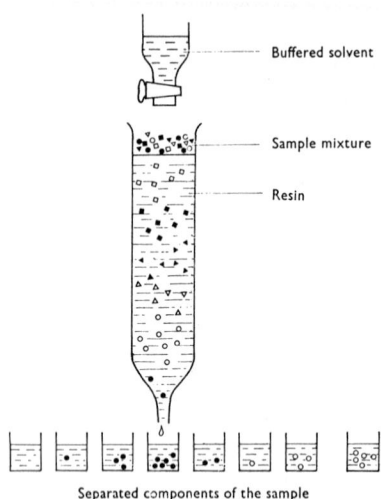

Separated components of the sample

Fig. 4.—The principle of column chromatography.

It is particularly important to use 'controls' in experimental work. Experiments, if they are to have any value, are almost always designed to test a hypothesis. In other words, the worker knows, or hopes he knows, the result he will obtain. Control experiments are designed to test the validity of the conclusions which might later be made from the results. Suppose we suspect, but do not know, that dentine contains nerves. Histological sections of dozens of teeth are prepared and stained in order to demonstrate nerve fibres. In one such series of studies in the 1930s the particular technique used seemed to show that every dentinal tubule contained nerve fibres. A control experiment could have taken the following form. In a group of animals, the inferior dental nerve would be cut and the animals

8

killed 2 or 3 weeks later. All the sensory nerve fibres in the lower teeth would have degenerated. If histological sections of these teeth had been prepared, it would have been found that all the dentinal tubules still contained nerve fibres. The 'controls' would have demonstrated that the stain was not picking out sensory nerve fibres from the inferior dental nerve, but probably staining the contents of dentinal tubules.

Finally, there is always the problem of correctly interpreting data. The classic example in this field is an experiment in which fleas were taught to jump on a word of command. It was found that if either of the two front pairs of legs was removed, fleas continued to jump on the word of command: but they did not respond if their back legs were removed. Evidently amputation of the hind legs leads to deafness in fleas. This is not an outrageous parody of scientific interpretations. It is by no means improbable that similar mistakes are made in the interpretation of many experiments, particularly those involving the analysis of complex biochemical systems which often involve unknown intermediate reactions.

CHAPTER 2

THE CELL

THE cell is the structural and functional unit of the living organism. Unicellular organisms have existed from the time of first life on earth and have colonized all known ecological niches. They must therefore be regarded as being highly 'successful'. However, it is the multicellular organisms that have provided the 'plastic' substrate upon which evolutionary processes have worked so dramatically. The increasing complexity of the multicellular organisms is still dependent upon the collective functioning of individual cells, each of which displays features common to all other cells in addition to features specific to its cell type.

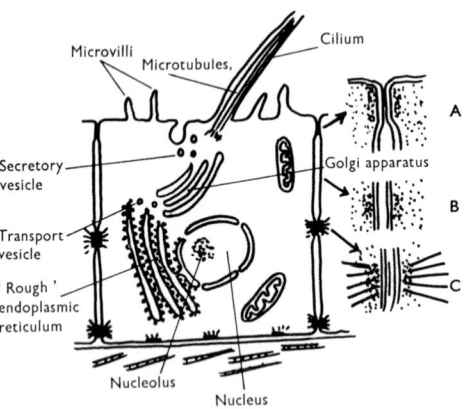

Fig. 5.—Diagrammatic representation of an epithelial cell as seen with the electron microscope. A, B, and C show higher detail of the zonula occludens, zonula adhaerens, and macula adhaerens (desmosome).

All cells contain certain components of distinctive size and shape, having a characteristic structure when viewed in the electron microscope and each contributing individually or collectively to the normal functioning of that cell: these components are termed 'organelles'. Most of the basic components of a cell are represented diagrammatically in *Figs.* 5 and 6. On the basis of electron microscopical studies, all organelles seen with the light microscope are now known to be formed on a skeleton of unit membranes. The membranous structures include the cell membrane, mitochondria,

Golgi apparatus, and endoplasmic reticulum, all of which have the same basic physical structure. Membrane components separate compartments such as the outside of the cell from the inside, or the contents of a vesicle from the cytoplasm; they also act as a surface for enzyme action, especially in mitochondria.

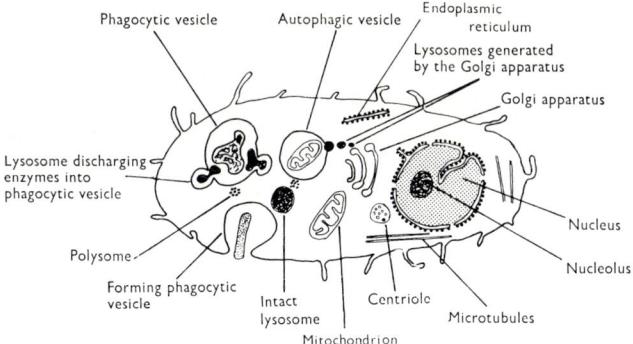

Fig. 6.—Diagram of cell showing components as they might appear under the electron microscope.

MEMBRANES

Structurally, unit membranes are generally considered to consist largely of a double chain of phospholipid molecules, each having a hydrophilic and a hydrophobic end. The hydrophilic groups line up along the outer surfaces of the double membrane and are bound, together with other lipid molecules, to proteins. The hydrophobic ends form the inside of the sandwich (*Fig. 7*). Although such a

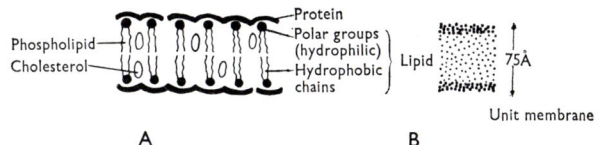

Fig. 7.—A, Diagram of structure of plasma membrane. B, Image of plasma membrane as seen in electron microscope section.

membrane is only 7–10 nm thick, it appears in electron micrographs of fixed cells as a distinct double line, which it is thought is due to the interaction between the fixative used and the protein and polar groups.

The above description of membranes is oversimplified because it relies too much on the appearance of membranes which have been distorted by fixation and dehydration in order that they can be viewed in the electron microscope. Studies of their activity suggest

11

that membranes consist of a lipid 'matrix', not necessarily homogeneous. Globular proteins, both enzyme and structural, may either be attached to the inside or outside of the membrane, or they may 'float' inside the lipid.

The function of membranes is to concentrate substances within, for example, a whole cell, a mitochondrion or a lysosome, thereby increasing the rate at which reactions can progress. Without membranes the contents of a cell would be diffused throughout its cytoplasm thereby reducing the rate at which potentially reactive components (e.g. an enzyme and its substrate) were brought together.

Different membranes 'capture' different globular proteins accounting for the different functions of each of the membranes shown in *Fig. 6*. The activity of the membrane may reflect the extent to which the proteins it has 'captured' lie on its surface or sink into its middle. In turn this may depend on the concentration of other substances in the surrounding cytoplasm. It was once remarked that so many different proteins have been described within the plasma membrane that there can be no room left for the membrane itself. But the proteins are as much a part of the membrane as the lipid which is stained by osmium and seen under the electron microscope.

The Plasma Membrane: Each cell is surrounded by a plasma membrane which forms a selective physical barrier between the cytoplasm and the extracellular compartment. Animal cell surfaces are nearly always irregular in shape with projections ranging in size from the large pseudo-podia extending from some mobile cells, to the very much smaller, specialized, finger-like microvilli and cilia of some epithelial cells (*Fig. 5*). In addition the plasma membrane may be invaginated to form pinocytotic vesicles containing fluid withdrawn from outside the cell, or phagocytic vesicles for the ingestion of more solid material (*Fig. 6*). Later in this chapter, when considering secretory cells and their functioning, it will be shown that substances produced within the cell often come to be contained within membranous vesicles which move to the cell periphery where they discharge their contents into the extracellular compartment by a process known as 'reverse pinocytosis'.

Contact between Cells: The surfaces of cells are charged and because adjacent similar cells have a similar surface charge their plasma membranes repel each other leaving a small 'space' between them. However, many cells, particularly epithelial cells, have specialized areas of the cell membrane by which they establish and maintain close contact with their neighbours. Three types of contact structures have been recognized in electron micrographs, viz. terminal bars (tight junctions or zonulae occludens), intermediate junctions (zonulae adhaerens), and desmosomes (maculae adhaerens).

12

Terminal bars are sited between cells towards their end furthest away from the basement membrane; here the electron-dense outer zones of adjacent cell membranes fuse and obliterate the intercellular space to form a continuous belt-like attachment. A band of electron-dense cytoplasm is found associated with this junction (*Fig. 5A*). Intermediate junctions are found between the cells midway along their length where the neighbouring cell membranes are closer together for a short distance though still separated by some homogeneous, amorphous material of low density; there are conspicuous bands of dense material in the adjacent cytoplasm (*Fig. 5B*). Desmosomes are present between cells proximal to the basement membrane at points where neighbouring cell membranes separate to generate a localized intercellular space approximately 24 nm wide. This space is filled with a button-like condensation of electron-dense material. Tonofibrils radiate out into the cytoplasm from associated areas of dense material (*Fig. 5*). Apart from providing intercellular attachments, it seems probable that desmosomes are regions through which material can, in some way, be passed from one cell to an adjacent cell.

Recently another type of cell-to-cell contact has been recognized. Although seemingly very similar to the tight junction in its morphology, it can be distinguished from the tight junction by demonstrating that an electron dense molecule (lanthanum) is able to pass between the two opposed plasma membranes, hence the term 'gap'. Gap junctions are thought to permit the transfer of 'information' between cells and to play an important role in differentiation.

THE NUCLEUS

Owing to the great affinity of the nucleus for histological stains it quickly became recognized as a component of all viable cells. Moreover, with improvements in the optical microscope and in staining techniques, coupled with the appreciation of its vital role in cell multiplication, the nucleus became almost the sole centre of cytological investigations for many years, the cytoplasm being largely neglected. The chromatin content of the nucleus and its relationship to the maintenance of cell lineage was quickly appreciated, but the precise mechanisms at work remained purely speculative until recent years. It then became known that the primary chemical substance of the genes was deoxyribonucleic acid (DNA), and furthermore that very large molecules composed of this DNA are responsible for carrying the specific information that enabled the cell to express its individuality. We now know that, apart from mitochondrial DNA and certain types of cells which appear to have small quantities in their cytoplasm, DNA is entirely located within the nucleus.

13

The nucleus of the cell is bounded by a double unit membrane containing numerous pores through which the contents of the nucleus are in contact with the cytoplasm. Within the nucleus are the chromosomes, which consist of very long double chains of DNA. Each long chain is subdivided into smaller units, the genes. The DNA is the master plan, in the form of templates, of all the activities of the body at the cellular level and every cell of one individual probably contains precisely the same set of templates.

The chromosomes are stabilized by attachments to the nuclear membrane.

DNA is 'naked' inert information expressed in one dimension— a linear sequence of nucleotides. Although convenient it is, strictly speaking, inaccurate to speak of DNA activity. The DNA can be exposed, it can be duplicated (during cell division) or its information can be copied in the form of RNA. But in each case the DNA is inactive: enzymes control and activate the above processes, working on the inert DNA.

Current theory indicates that the functional state of a cell is the result of the activity of the DNA of that cell. For example, a part of the genetic information contained in the DNA may become permanently blocked and therefore rendered ineffective and this represents a permanent change in that cell; in other words the cell has differentiated. Alternatively, parts of the DNA chain may be selectively activated or suppressed, depending on the functional requirements of the cell, and this change is a reversible one. There-fore, in terms of function, cells differ solely in which parts of the plans they use. Thus a fibroblast can be distinguished because it makes use of those parts of the DNA chain which contain the plans for collagen formation, an ameloblast those parts concerned with enamel matrix formation. However, the master plans (DNA) remain almost exclusively within the nucleus and only copies of the relevant parts of them are carried into the cytoplasm by means of a form of ribonucleic acid known as 'messenger' ribonucleic acid ('messenger' RNA), which is manufactured on the templates of the DNA in the nucleus.

Experimental procedures involving the injection of radioactive inorganic phosphate into animal tissues, whereby the RNA molecule is labelled, show the initial labelling only in the nucleolus. Only with the passing of time is there labelling of the cytoplasmic RNA. These and similar results strongly suggest that RNA is only synthe-sized in the nucleus, whence the molecules migrate into the cyto-plasm. 'Messenger' RNA may thus be regarded as the co-ordinating agent between nucleus and cytoplasm. More refined techniques suggest, however, that there may also be some RNA synthesis in the cytoplasm, but as yet the evidence is rather inconclusive.

14

The nucleolus is particularly involved in the production of 'ribo-somal' RNA (*see below*).

The relationship between nucleus and cytoplasm has been elegantly demonstrated by removing the nuclei from single-celled animals (protozoa). These experiments show that the cell is only capable of performing all its functions when nucleus and cytoplasm are in mutual coexistence.

The above account leads to the conclusion that the function of the nucleus is twofold. It contains the DNA which is responsible for the maintenance of cell lineage, although it must be remembered that recognizable chromosomes containing the DNA are only visible during mitosis. This same DNA is in reality the coded information which, during the life span of the cell, is passed to those centres of the cytoplasm whose function is to control the synthesis and release of selected proteins required at any one moment.

PROTEIN SYNTHESIS

Under the light microscope the cytoplasm of the living cell seems to consist of a clear, colourless material within which countless opaque particles are in constant, apparently random, movement. The electron microscope reveals even more structures (organelles) within the cytoplasm of the fixed cell. In many cells the organelles for protein synthesis are prominent; these consist of ribosomes composed of a second form of RNA and the associated endoplasmic reticulum (*see below*). It will be recalled that 'messenger' RNA is synthesized within the nucleus on the templates of DNA. From here, the 'messenger' RNA carries its information, also in the form of templates, to cytoplasmic aggregations of 'ribosomal' RNA where protein is synthesized by joining together amino-acids.

The bonds connecting amino-acids in a polypeptide chain do not form spontaneously; when amino-acids are mixed in a test-tube no linkage occurs. For linkage to occur energy is required. Energy in the form of adenosine triphosphate (ATP) is donated enzymatically within the cell and the amino-acid is spoken of as being 'activated'. The activated amino-acids are brought to the ribosome by one of a series of 'transfer' or soluble RNA molecules (the third form of RNA) each of which is specific for a particular amino-acid. In the ribosome the 'transfer' RNA molecules, with their attached activated amino-acids, take their appropriate places on the template so that the amino-acids are aligned and held in proper sequence to form a specific polypeptide chain. The complex of 'ribosomal' 'messenger' RNA, and 'transfer' RNA, plus the forming polypeptide chain, together constitute the polysome. A good analogy here is the auto-mated machine tool. The ribosome represents the machine tool, the 'messenger' RNA the tape with its coded instructions, and the 'transfer' RNA is the conveyor belt bringing the raw materials.

DNA consists of information for the sequence of amino-acids in every protein produced by the body. But the specific shape of a globular protein is determined by its environment. And it is these proteins (structural and enzyme) which organize the shape of a mitochondrion, a cell, an organ, a limb, and an animal itself.

Endoplasmic Reticulum and Golgi Apparatus: It appears that there are two main paths of protein production: one for the replacement of cell components or for retention within the cell, the other for the synthesis of protein for secretion from the cell. Protein for internal use is produced by ribosomes distributed within the cytoplasm most frequently in groups forming 'rosettes' (*Fig. 8*). Cells which undergo

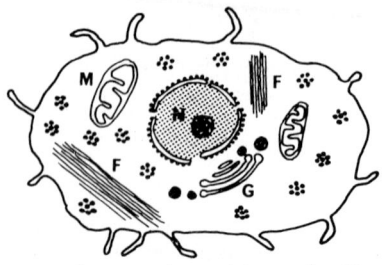

Fig. 8.—Diagram of a protein-retaining cell. Note the poorly formed Golgi apparatus (G), evenly scattered 'rosettes', and absence of rough membranes. F, Retained protein fibres; M, Mitochondrion; N, Nucleolus in the nucleus.

keratinization are of this type, having evenly distributed 'rosettes', a simple and relatively insignificant Golgi apparatus, and a demonstrably increasing number of retained protein filaments in their cytoplasm (*Fig. 8*). In cells such as mucous cells and ameloblasts where proteins are produced for secretion the mechanism is slightly different. Here the ribosomes are associated with the surface of the endoplasmic reticulum which is composed of a series of flattened interconnected vesicles, giving the reticulum a 'rough' appearance in electron micrographs (*Fig. 5*). The protein synthesized on the ribosomes passes into the lumen of this 'rough' endoplasmic reticulum and may be secreted directly from there.

More commonly the products pass from the 'rough' endoplasmic reticulum into the lumen of the 'smooth' endoplasmic reticulum (so called on account of the absence of associated ribosomes) or Golgi apparatus (*Fig. 5*). As more and more of the secretory material accumulates the 'smooth' endoplasmic reticulum swells and buds off to form discrete secretory vesicles. In the pancreas, for example, the secretory vesicles contain the pancreatic enzymes, or in goblet cells the secretion is mucus. Gradually the secretory vesicles move to the free border of the cell where their encompassing membrane fuses with the cell membrane, a break appears in the cell surface and the contents of the vesicle are extruded from the cell by a secretory vesicle (*Fig. 5*). Recent work has shown that the Golgi apparatus is not just a series of passively distensible sacs but that it can modify the proteins passing through by attaching carbohydrates to them.

Lysosomes

The Golgi apparatus is also concerned with the production of lysosomes. These cytoplasmic bodies (*Fig. 6*) are concentrations of active hydrolytic enzymes surrounded by a single membrane. There are more than twenty lysosomal enzymes and they are all active at an acid pH. Lysosomal enzymes are found in the Golgi apparatus and lysosomes are formed by the pinching off of small vesicles from the edges of the Golgi saccules (*Fig. 6*). When a human macrophage or a phagocytic animal like an amoeba ingests solid material, tissue debris, or an organism, a phagocytic vesicle is formed (*Fig. 6*). Cytoplasmic lysosomes fuse with this vesicle, their enzymes are discharged into it, and the contained phagocytosed material is broken down.

In addition to the breakdown of material in phagocytic vesicles, lysosomal enzymes are employed to break down damaged or unwanted organelles like mitochondria. This takes place in 'autophagic' vesicles. The organelle is first isolated from the cytoplasm by a membrane thereby forming a vesicle into which lysosomal enzymes are injected. In this way the cell is able selectively to eliminate single organelles without digesting other cytoplasmic components.

MITOCHONDRIA AND ENERGY PRODUCTION

Processes such as protein synthesis and other functions performed by cells require energy. This energy is mainly derived from the breakdown of high-energy phosphate compounds such as adenosine triphosphate (ATP); mitochondria are the main sources of ATP production. The cytoplasm of all living cells, except bacteria and mature red blood cells, contains numerous mitochondria. They may vary considerably in outline but all have an outer limiting membrane within which there is an additional membrane, infolded to produce a pattern of cristae that serve to increase the surface area of the interior for catalytic purposes. Most recent work shows that mitochondria divide and grow, rather than arising *de novo*, or from non-mitochondrial precursors.

Highly refined biochemical techniques have shown that the mitochondria contain numerous enzymes. Some of these enzymes are concerned with the Krebs cycle. This involves the progressive oxidation of a succession of organic acids, each stage being governed by a different and specific enzyme. At various parts of the cycle energy is generated and CO_2 is released. This is a true cycle in that the starting substrate is reconstituted at the end and is ready to re-run the cycle provided the requisite enzyme is available. Much of the energy produced in the mitochondria is used to reconstitute ATP. This substance is used in various processes in many parts of the cell, for when it is broken down it releases the energy again. The mitochondria may thus be regarded as centres of energy production within the cell, in fact they are the 'power house' of the cell.

MICROTUBULES

A group of intracellular structures whose importance has only recently been recognized is the microtubular system. These microtubules (*Figs. 5* and *6*) may be several μm in length, typically 25 nm in diameter, and have an electron dense wall which under the highest powers of magnification contains a number of filamentous units, the central core being appreciably less electron dense, though it is doubtful whether it is patent. The tubules show no evidence of branching, are remarkably straight, and available evidence shows them to be stiff and elastic with a high tendency to return to the straight form after distortion. Microtubules appear to perform three main functions. First, they arise from the centrioles during cell division and provide the spindle along which the chromosomes separate. Second, sheaths of the tubules form the motile element of cilia and flagella and, third, microtubules play a role in the transport of substances through cytoplasm. In connexion with the latter function it is significant that they are particularly prominent in cells with long processes such as odontoblasts and neurons where the extremities of the cell may be a very long way from the nuclear region.

Finally, cells contain numerous microfilaments which appear to be able to contract, thereby distorting the cell. For example, when the cytoplasm of a cell splits at the end of mitosis, microfilaments are arranged circumferentially around the equator along which the cell divides. It is possible that the equatorial furrow in the surface of the dividing cell is produced by contraction of the underlying microfilaments.

BASEMENT LAMINA AND MEMBRANE

For many years light microscopists have recognized that the layer of extracellular tissue separating epithelial from mesodermal cells stains heavily with silver. This layer consists of collagen fibres and ground substance and is referred to as the 'basement membrane'. Its activity in maintaining the viability of epithelial cells, and in mediating those elements which induce the differentiation of epithelial cells, will be referred to in a later chapter.

The basement membrane of the light microscope is more complex when seen in the electron microscope. The layer of collagen fibres is referred to as the 'reticular lamina'. With the magnifications that can be achieved with electron microscopy another structure is visible between the reticular lamina and the plasma membranes of the epithelial cells. This is called the 'basement lamina'. The basement lamina consists of a clear (lamina lucida) and a dense (lamina densa) layer. Because it is so thin (about 100 nm thick) it has not been possible to characterize the substances contained in the basement lamina.

We have so far described the structure and functioning of the cell in isolation, but in the multicellular animal relatively few cells exist in isolation. The multicellular grade of organization confers upon an animal a great variety of advantages over its unicellular ancestor not the least of which is the great potential for evolutionary changes developing in such cellular agglomerations. The setting aside of certain groups of cells, some to perform one and some another function for the good of the entire animal, is the process by which tissues and organs evolve. These are but steps in the process of cell and tissue differentiation and the establishment of the division of labour within the multicellular organism.

We have seen that, apart from viruses, the cell forms the fundamental unit of all living matter and whatever their ultimate function all cells are but modifications of a basic type. We have briefly touched upon the concept of the tissue and of the organ, wherein intercellular co-operation permits functional specialization and division of labour, the advent of which is recognized as being a step of fundamental importance in the evolution of progressive forms of animal life. Within the remaining chapters of this book the concept of functional specialization of the cell will be extended and developed in so far as it is concerned with the production of the definitive human tooth.

REFERENCES

Butler J. A. V. (1959) *Inside the Living Cell.* London, Allen & Unwin.
Chedd G. (1968) 'Ribosomes: The Assembly Shops of Life—1', *New Scient.* **39,** No. 607, 175.
Chedd G. (1968) 'Ribosomes: The Assembly Shops of Life—2', *New Scient.* **39,** No. 608, 233.

Farquhar M. G. and Palade G. E. (1963) Junctional complexes in various epithelia. *J. Cell Biol.* **17,** 375.

Jacob F. and Monod J. (1961) Genetic regulatory mechanisms in the synthesis of proteins, *J. Mol. Biol.* **3,** 318.

'The Living Cell' (1965) In: *Readings from Scientific American.* San Francisco, Freeman.

Loewy A. G. and Siekevitz R. (1963) *Cell Structure and Function.* London, Holt, Rinehart & Winston.

Mercer E. H. (1963) *Cells and Cell Structure.* London, Hutchinson.

Neutra M. and Leblond C. P. (1969) The Golgi apparatus. *Sci. Am.* **220,** 100.

Porter K. R. (1966) Cytoplasmic microtubules and their functions. In: Wolstenholme G. E. W. and O'Connor J. (ed.), *Principles of Bimolecular Organization.* London, Churchill.

CHAPTER 3

THE TOOTH IN SITU

THIS brief description of the developing and completed human tooth in situ is meant to introduce the student to the terminology and position of the salient tissues as they might appear in a section of a human jaw. The composite diagrams in *Figs. 9* and *10* provide a glossary of components rather than an accurate histological picture. The boxed numbers appearing alongside some of the structures and tissues labelled in *Fig. 10* refer to the chapter in this book dealing specifically with the features in question, so that the diagrams may also serve as a rapid index.

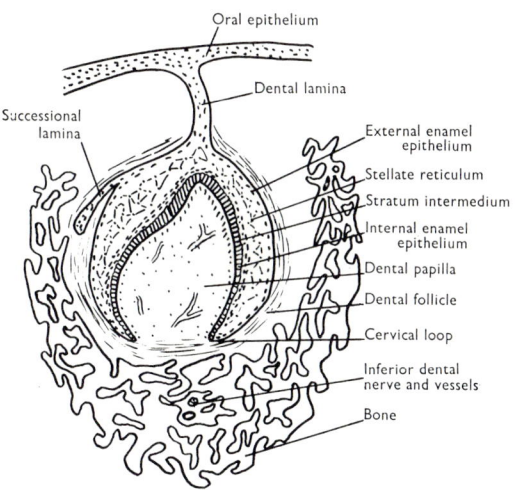

Fig. 9.—Diagram of a section of a developing tooth in situ.

The forming tooth germ (*Fig. 9*) has reached the bell stage of development, during which tissues concerned with crown production are rapidly differentiating.

The enamel organ comprises an outer enamel epithelium which is continuous with the basal layer of the oral epithelium via the dental lamina. At the cervical loop the outer enamel epithelium folds sharply and continues over the surface of the papilla as the inner enamel epithelium. Adjacent to the inner enamel epithelium, and within the enamel organ, is a layer of stratified cells forming

21

the stratum intermedium. The enamel organ is occupied by a diffuse stellate reticulum which is largely composed of intercellular fluid-filled spaces.

The richly vascular dental papilla contains the many types of cells found in any connective tissue. Its surface is lined by odontoblasts whose chief function is to produce dentine.

Each tooth germ is separated from the alveolar bone by its own fibrous tooth follicle which expands as the tooth grows.

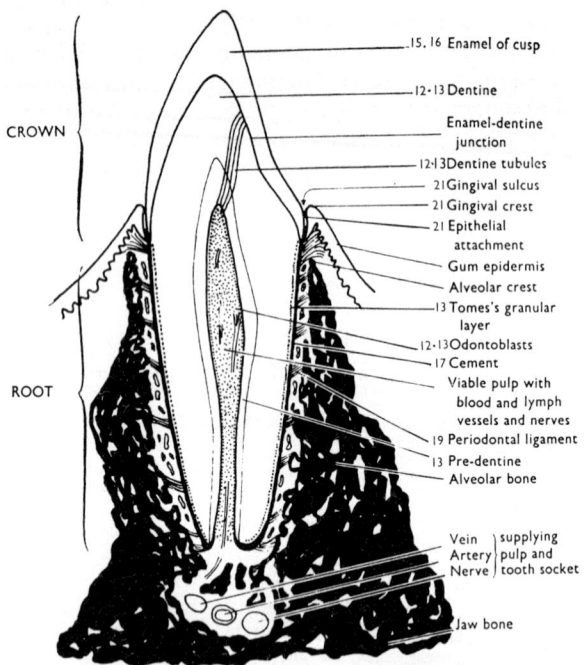

CROWN

ROOT

.15, 16 Enamel of cusp

12-13 Dentine

Enamel-dentine junction

12-13 Dentine tubules

21 Gingival sulcus

21 Gingival crest

21 Epithelial attachment

Gum epidermis

Alveolar crest

13 Tomes's granular layer

12-13 Odontoblasts

17 Cement

Viable pulp with blood and lymph vessels and nerves

19 Periodontal ligament

13 Pre-dentine

Alveolar bone

Vein ⎫ supplying
Artery ⎬ pulp and
Nerve ⎭ tooth socket

Jaw bone

Fig. 10.—Composite diagram of a longitudinal section of a functional tooth in situ.

On the lingual side of the tooth germ, in the region of its attachment to the dental lamina, a successional lamina develops at whose deep edge grows the germ of the permanent tooth.

The nerve and vascular supplies to the tooth germ are derived from main trunks lying beneath its base.

The completed and functional tooth (*Fig. 10*) consists of an enamel covered anatomical crown and a cement-covered anatomical root. The term 'anatomical crown' must be distinguished from the term 'clinical crown'. The clinical crown is that part of the tooth which is exposed in the mouth at any given age. In young persons part of the base of the anatomical crown remains hidden by the gingival margin so that the clinical crown is smaller than the anatomical crown. In elderly persons the gingival margin retreats rootwards (passive eruption), exposing the entire anatomical crown and also often a small portion of the anatomical root. The clinical crown is now larger than the anatomical crown.

The anatomical root is all that part of the tooth lying deep to the level of the cervical margin of the enamel and typically contained within the bony alveolus (socket). Enamel is not normally present on the root except as enamel droplets, commonly found in the root bifurcations of molars.

By far the greatest proportion of a tooth consists of dentine, a mineralized tissue permeated throughout its thickness by regularly arranged dentine tubules, each containing a fine protoplasmic process of an odontoblast cell which is itself situated on the surface of the pulp. The outer surface of the coronal dentine lines the enamel-dentine junction which is microscopically irregular. A further mineralized tissue, cement, lies on the outer surface of the root and serves as an attachment for fibres of the periodontal ligament (*see below*). Immediately beneath the surface of the root dentine there is a microscopically granular layer, termed the 'granular layer of Tomes'. In the centre of the coronal dentine is the pulp chamber which in a young tooth extends as a pulp horn beneath the cusp. A pulp canal runs the entire length of each root and opens into the periodontal ligament at the apical foramen. The tissue within the pulp cavity is a normal connective tissue covered by specialized cells, the odontoblasts.

Enamel is the refractile microcrystalline, highly mineralized layer on the outer surface of the anatomical crown.

The only site where oral epithelium comes into direct contact with the functional tooth is at the base of the clinical crown. Here the epithelium is turned inwards and attached to the surface of the enamel, producing the gingival sulcus and the epithelial attachment.

The tooth is anchored to its socket in the alveolar bone by the collagen fibres of the periodontal ligament. Most of these fibres run obliquely and coronally from the cement into the alveolar bone. The bundles of fibres which are inserted into the mineralized tissues are called 'Sharpey's fibres'. The term 'alveolar bone' refers to that part of the jaw which contains holes (alveoli). It is not in any way histologically distinguishable from the remaining bone tissue of the jaws. It exists solely to support the teeth and is largely resorbed when the teeth are lost.

CHAPTER 4

THE ROLE OF ECTOMESENCHYME IN TOOTH FORMATION AND INDUCTION

THE neural crest, which is the source of ectomesenchyme, is an important primordium found in the early embryo. The fertilized egg rapidly develops to form an embryonic disk consisting of two cell types, an outer layer of ectoderm and an inner layer of endoderm. The space between these two germ layers comes to be occupied by a third germ layer, the mesoderm, thus establishing the trilaminar embryo. At this time the longitudinal axis of the embryo is emphasized by the formation of the neural plate, a symmetrical demarcated area of ectoderm, wider at the future head end, bounded by thickened marginal folds, and extending along the future dorsal surface (*Fig. 11*). In time the neural folds rise up and, approaching each other,

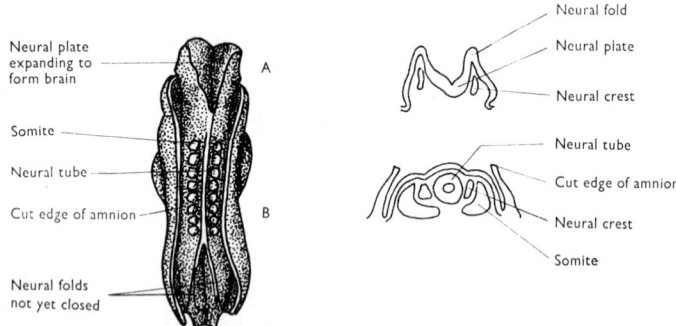

Fig. 11.—Dorsal view of human embryo of 2·1 mm showing developing central nervous system. To the right, diagrammatic cross-sections at levels A and B.

meet and fuse along the midline, thus converting the neural plate into a tube which sinks inwards beneath the surface ectoderm. During the development of the neural tube small groups of ecto-dermal cells break away from the margins of the neural plate and come to lie parallel to, and on either side of, the neural tube. These constitute the neural crest cells. The mesoderm gives rise to embryonic connective tissue or mesenchyme (mesodermal mesenchyme) from which differentiates a wide range of cells and tissues such as fibrous tissue, adipose tissue, tendons and ligaments. The neural crest is the source of a tremendous variety of cell and tissue types:

pigment cells, Schwann cells, the meninges of the brain, the cells of the spinal and autonomic ganglia, the adrenal medulla and large amounts of mesenchyme (called either 'mesectoderm' or 'ectomesenchyme'). Much of the branchial arch mesenchyme is derived from this source.

The refined techniques of experimental embryology have extended our knowledge of the role of neural crest far beyond the limitations associated with the examination of serial sections of normal embryo. Much of this work, involving delicate ablation, extirpation, and transplantation of neural crest tissue, has been performed on larval forms of fish and amphibia and also on chick embryos. In some of these animals the neural crest cells are pigmented or are laden with yolk particles, differing from the yolk-free surrounding cells, which enable them to be traced for some time in sections of the embryos. Marking such cells with *intra-vitam* dyes, or more recently with radioactively labelled compounds, greatly increases the ease with which their migratory routes can be followed during development.

The collective information obtained from these experiments shows without doubt that, in the early developing stages of these vertebrates, the branchial arch cartilages from which the jaws arise are formed from ectomesenchyme which has migrated downwards from near the mid-dorsal line. Moreover, while the formation of the mouth depends upon the inductive interaction between ectoderm and endoderm, no teeth develop on jaws unless ectomesenchyme is also present. De Beer (1947) was able to show conclusively that the odontoblasts of larval salamander teeth are of ectomesenchymal origin, and that in this animal some of the enamel organs may be of ectodermal and others of endodermal origin. Hence he concluded that ectomesenchyme is the primary factor in inducing the formation of the enamel organ from the overlying surface epithelium, irrespective of its origin from ectoderm or endoderm.

Experiments on mammalian embryos comparable with those on amphibian larvae are not so easily undertaken. However, recent experiments on rat embryos maintained in organ culture, in which the migration of neural crest cells has been studied by labelling them with radioisotopes, have shown that the findings made on amphibian and avian embryos can be applied to mammals. Other indirect evidence is also available. It is well established that in very early embryos areas of morphogenesis tend to be rich in RNA, and that gradients of RNA concentration signify gradients of morphogenetic or metabolic activity. Furthermore, areas of morphogenesis are also rich in alkaline phosphatase activity and glycogen. These properties have been used to observe, in closely timed serial sections of mouse embryos, ectomesenchyme streaming into the maxillary

25

and mandibular processes (*Fig. 12*) where it amasses beneath the surface ectoderm, at a time before the latter shows any evidence of the thickening which is generally recognized as the initial stage of tooth formation.

It is now widely recognized that in addition to having high concentrations of RNA, alkaline phosphatase and glycogen, regions of intense morphogenesis are also the sites of vascular concentration. In the embryo cat, which has been closely studied, the capillary

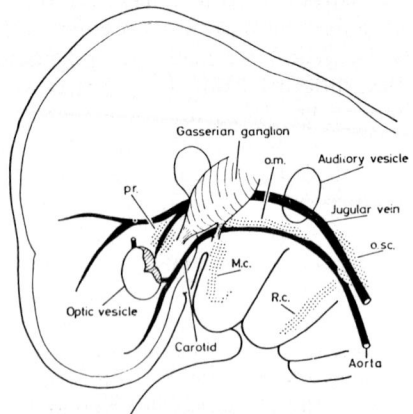

Fig. 12.—Diagram showing the distribution of mesenchyme rich in alkaline phosphatase (stippled) in the head region of a 10-day mouse embryo. Vessels supplying the branchial arches are omitted. M.c., precursor of Meckel's cartilage; o.m., primordium of external rectus muscle; o.sc., occipital sclerotomes; pr., premandibular area; R.c., precursor of Reichert's cartilage. (*Reproduced from Milaire J.*, 1959, *Archs Biol.*, *Liège*, **70**, 587.)

vascular system within the mesenchyme underlying the future position of the tooth germs is established before there is any evidence of the epithelial thickening associated with the dental lamina. Even at a slightly later stage, the capillary density increases in relation to the dental lamina at the sites of future tooth germs, before corresponding epithelial activity. Hence, it is possible to predict the location of the tooth buds and of diastemata by observing the distribution of capillary density along the length of the jaw.

It must be apparent to the reader that none of these observations is related specifically to the human embryo. However, there is no reason to think that other mammalian embryos are radically different from the human embryo in their development.

From the above evidence it is clear that ectomesenchyme plays an important role in the organization of the tissues of the vertebrate

26

jaws, including the teeth. However, it would be unwise to state that the ectomesenchyme has the sole responsibility for inducing the development of the ectodermal component of the tooth. During the past few years a great deal of work has been done on epithelial-mesenchymal interactions by separating them with an inert membrane specially manufactured for such studies. With this technique epithelium and mesenchyme are first separated and then *in vitro* brought together on either side of the inert membrane. Using this technique, mesenchyme from one source can be brought close to epithelium taken from a different site in the body and the effects of one on the other studied. Thus, presumptive salivary mesenchyme (mesenchyme which will later become incorporated as the supporting tissue of a salivary gland) with presumptive salivary epithelium induces the differentiation of glandular salivary epithelium. In contrast, ordinary jaw mesenchyme is unable to induce the differentiation of glandular salivary epithelium, but it will prevent the presumptive salivary epithelium from degenerating. Finally, presumptive pancreatic epithelium associated with salivary gland mesenchyme differentiates into pancreatic gland cells.

The above experiments suggest the existence of three types of epithelial/mesenchymal relations. First, epithelium requires a 'mesodermal maintenance factor' without which it will degenerate. Second, some mesenchyme can induce epithelia from a variety of sites to differentiate into a tissue 'dictated' by the mesenchyme. Third, some apparently undifferentiated epithelia are in fact differentiated and mesenchyme is only capable of triggering the final overt stages of differentiation; the mesenchyme cannot 'dictate' the direction in which the epithelium differentiates.

Not only does the mesenchyme induce epithelium, but the epithelium also acts back on the mesenchyme. Thus, it is clear that the histogenesis of a complex structure such as the tooth is the result of an obligatory interaction between mesenchyme and epidermal tissues. Whilst it is appreciated that such interaction exists, the mechanism whereby information is passed from one tissue to another is not understood. The developing tooth is being used as a model system to study this problem and some possibly significant information is being obtained. The assumption is made that, during epithelial mesenchymal interactions, cells synthesize molecules which are transferred to the extracellular matrix where they may act on adjacent cells. Extracellular matrix, freed of its cellular components, has been examined in the developing tooth at the time of initial dentinogenesis (the differentiation of odontoblasts is induced by epithelial cells) and found to contain vesicular structures, some of which might contain ribonucleic acid. Whilst ribonucleic acid would provide an ideal vehicle for the passage of information, only its

27

presence, not its actual transfer between epithelial and mesenchymal cells, has been demonstrated.

REFERENCES

De Beer G. R. (1947) The differentiation of neural crest cells into odontoblasts in ambystoma and re-examination of the germ-layer theory. *Proc. R. Soc.* **134-B,** 377.

Fleischmajer R. and Billingham R. E. (1968) *Epithelial-Mesenchymal Interactions.* Baltimore, Williams & Wilkins.

Gaunt W. A. (1959) The vascular supply to the dental lamina during early development. *Acta Anat.* **37,** 232.

Gaunt W. A. and Miles A. E. W. (1967) Fundamental aspects of tooth morphogenesis. In: Miles A. E. W. (ed.), *Structural and Chemical Organization of Teeth*, vol. 1. New York, Academic.

Kollar E. J. and Baird G. R. (1970) Tissue interactions in embryonic mouse tooth germs. *J. Emb. exp. Morph.* **24,** 159.

Kollar E. J. and Baird G. R. (1970) Tissue interactions in embryonic mouse tooth germs. *J. Emb. exp. Morph.* **24,** 173.

Slavkin H. C. (1974) Embryonic tooth formation. In: Melcher A. H. and Zarb G. A. (ed.), *Oral Sciences Reviews*, vol. 4. Copenhagen, Munskgaard.

Slavkin H. C. and Bavetta L. A. (1972) *Developmental Aspects of Oral Biology.* New York, Academic.

CHAPTER 5

THE EARLY DEVELOPMENT OF THE TEETH

IT is not intended to give here a detailed account of the histological changes which have been observed during development of the human tooth. The reader is referred to standard texts for complete details.

The epithelium in the front of the definitive mouth is derived from the lining of the original invaginated stomatodeum and is accordingly of ectodermal origin. Further back in the mouth the oral lining is derived from the endoderm of the embryonic pharynx, though the precise line of demarcation is a point of controversy (*Fig. 13*).

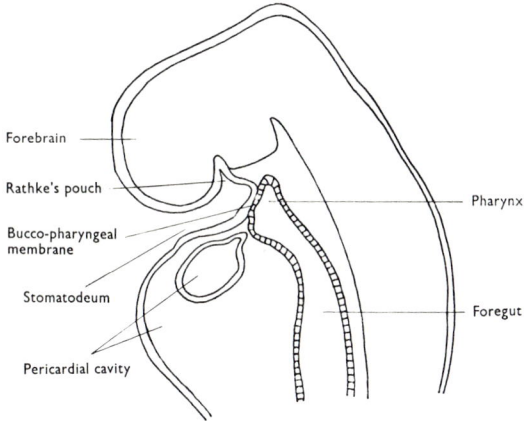

Forebrain

Rathke's pouch

Pharynx

Bucco-pharyngeal
membrane

Stomatodeum

Foregut

Pericardial cavity

Fig. 13.—Diagrammatic sagittal section of the head of 2.5-mm human embryo. Tissue of endodermal origin is cross-hatched.

Certainly, there is no detectable histological distinction to be seen in tissue sections taken through regions where the bucco-pharyngeal membrane has broken down.

At the time of initiation of the processes which will result in tooth formation, the potential tooth-bearing areas and the lips are covered by a considerably thicker layer of epithelial cells than the remainder of the primitive pharynx. These cells are rich in glycogen but, because glycogen is lost in the normal preparation of tissues for histological sectioning, the cells may appear vacuolated.

Studies of closely timed series of mouse embryos show that the first indication of the processes which will result in tooth formation

29

consists of a condensation of ectomesenchyme tissue immediately beneath the surface epithelium, along the tooth-bearing region of each jaw (*Fig. 14A*). The condensation first appears at the front

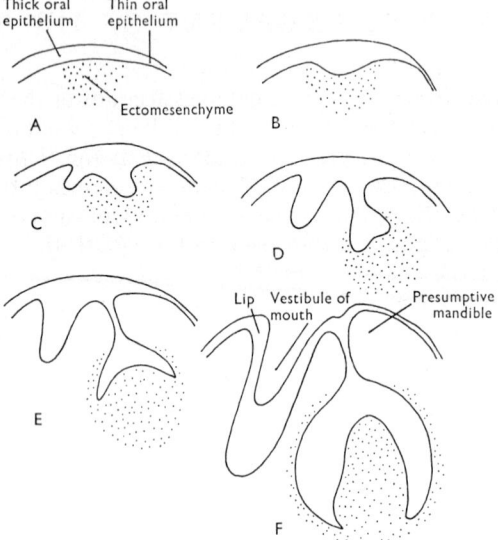

Fig. 14.—Each diagram represents a sagittal section of the skull through the subsequent incisor region.

A, Ectomesenchyme is concentrated beneath the thick pharyngeal epithelium which covers the subsequent tooth bearing region of the jaw. The lip will be to the left. B, the formation of the primary epithelial band. C, The vestibular band pushes anteriorly into the adjacent mesenchyme while the dental lamina grows into the ectomesenchyme. D, A tooth bud forms at the end of the dental lamina. The vestibular band increases in size. E, The ectodermal part of the tooth bud extends around the growing ball of ectomesenchymal cells to produce a cap. F, Continued growth of the ectodermal cells around the growing ball of ectomesenchymal cells results in a bell-shaped enamel organ. The central cells of the vestibular band break down separating a lip on the left from the subsequent alveolar region of the jaw on the right.

of the mouth, close to the midline, and spreads steadily backwards along each jaw quadrant, that in the lower jaw being slightly in advance of the upper. The precocity of the developmental processes in the lower jaw persists throughout ontogeny. This condensation of ectomesenchyme is probably responsible for the primary inductive influence in tooth formation referred to in the previous chapter. However, blood-capillaries are more numerous in the region of the ectomesenchymal condensation than in other regions of the jaws.

Following closely on this the oral epithelium adjacent to the ectomesenchyme begins to proliferate and protrudes into the underlying cellular condensation (*Fig. 14B*). The epithelial prominence is referred to as the 'primary epithelial band'. The position of the primary epithelial band may be controlled by a prior genetic determination of either the position at which the ectomesenchyme condenses, or by the sprouting of capillary networks, or by both. Frequent references are made in textbooks of embryology to the unbroken continuity of the primary epithelial band across the midline of the developing mammalian jaw. However, recent work shows quite clearly that in mouse, cat, and human embryos the band develops individually in each jaw quadrant, only uniting in the midline anteriorly in the 15 mm C.R. stage human embryo.

At this stage the primary epithelial band is shaped like a horseshoe (more accurately, a catenary), following the outline of the subsequent dental arcade. While continuing to proliferate into the ectomesenchyme the primary epithelial band starts pushing a buccal extension into the adjacent mesenchyme (*Fig. 14C*). The former extension is now referred to as the 'dental lamina' and the buccal extension as the 'vestibular lamina'.

Standard textbook descriptions imply that the dental lamina progressively invades the underlying ectomesenchyme so that as individual tooth germs bud from it they progressively come to lie deeper within the jaw. However, an alternative explanation seems possible. Namely, that on each side of the dental lamina the ectomesenchymal cells proliferate and push the oral epithelium towards the cavity of the pharynx away from the developing tooth germs, stretching the connexion (the dental lamina) between them. When, in later developmental stages, the lamina breaks down, severing this connexion, it appears to be split apart in tissue sections, an appearance which accords well with the above suggestion.

The ectomesenchymal cells adjacent to the growing end of the dental lamina now appear to clump in regions which correspond with those of the subsequent tooth germs. Just as in the earlier stages of tooth development when the whole dental lamina proliferated into the ectomesenchyme, so at this later stage, following the regional clumping of ectomesenchyme, stalks of dental lamina continue proliferating into the now localized condensations. These stalks and the adjacent ectomesenchyme are the tooth buds (*Fig. 14D*).

The above account of the differentiation of the earliest tooth buds is the one most usually given. However, there is an alternative interpretation of the microscopical appearances seen in tissue sections of these very early human embryos.

Some workers consider that the dental and vestibular laminar arise separately from the oral epithelium and that there is no such structure as the primary epithelial band. Reference to *Fig 14B* and

31

C, which illustrate the typical appearances of the relevant stages, show that it is quite possible that the vestibular lamina has a separate origin to that of the dental lamina. Indeed, in some animals, such as the crocodile, the first teeth develop from the oral mucosa without any obvious dental lamina having been formed.

The ectomesenchymal cells continue to proliferate thereby increasing the size of the ball of cells adjacent to the epithelial part of the tooth bud. But the epithelium itself continues to proliferate in what might be described as an attempt to surround the growing ball of ectomesenchymal cells. Some of the ectomesenchymal cells become pushed aside and are to be found around the edges of the encircling epithelial cells. The encircling attempts are 'more successful' and the epithelium spreads out to form a cap of cells on top of the ectomesenchyme (*Fig. 14E*). This is the cap stage of tooth development. It is during this stage that histo-differentiation begins, the definitive tissues of the dental organ differentiating, each to play

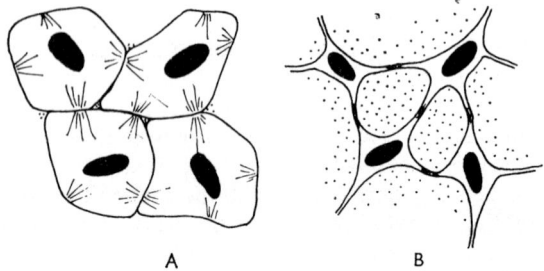

A   B

Fig. 15.—A, Four polygonal cells within the centre of the enamel organ secrete mucopolysaccharides (stippled) into the intercellular region. The mucopolysaccharides are hydrophilic and water is absorbed (B). The desmosomal connexions between the cells are maintained producing the stellate reticulum.

a specific role in the generation of the completed tooth. As the epithelial cap grows its central cells become increasingly separated from the vascular ectomesenchyme. The innermost cells begin to secrete acidic mucopolysaccharides into the narrow intercellular spaces separating them (*Fig. 15*). The mucopolysaccharides are intensely hydrophilic and water is pulled into the intercellular spaces, compressing the cytoplasm of each of the cells within the inner mass. All the cells of the enamel organ are united by desmosomes and despite the compression of their cytoplasm the desmosomal connexions between the inner cells are maintained. This process results in the development of a stellate reticulum whose intercellular spaces are filled with water and mucopolysaccharides.

Owing to the appearance of intercellular fluid-filled spaces the stellate reticulum swells into a turgid diffuse tissue whose functions may be considered under two headings, mechanical and nutritional. In a mechanical sense, it has been suggested that the stellate reticulum serves to protect the developing tooth germ against mechanical disturbance from without, and also to provide the requisite space for crown development within the tooth follicle. It has also been suggested that the tissue's turgor pressure serves to maintain the spherical shape of the dental organ during development and at the same time to balance the growth pressures generated by the expanding dental papilla (ectomesenchyme).

Early workers believed that the stellate reticulum provided a source of inorganic salts or ions to be drawn upon for enamel formation. However, neither histochemical nor micro-incineration techniques have revealed an abnormally high calcium content in the stellate reticulum either before or during the phase of enamel formation. The stellate reticulum is, however, rich in acidic mucopolysaccharide which generally diminishes during enamel formation. The provision of this substance may well be its main nutritive role.

The epithelial cells adjacent to the ectomesenchyme become cuboidal and then low columnar in shape, the layer being now called the 'inner enamel epithelium'. The cells of the outer enamel epithelium remain roughly cuboidal.

At this time the centre of the inner enamel epithelium is swollen into a mass of cells comprising the enamel knot. Workers in the early part of the nineteenth century attached great importance to this transitory structure believing it acted as a stable 'nucleus' of form-determining function. Closely associated with the knot is a cellular condensation traversing the stellate reticulum to unite with the outer enamel epithelium close to the latter's attachment to the dental lamina. This enamel cord, which may later thicken to become a septum, could contribute cells to the stellate reticulum.

The outer enamel epithelium plays a passive role in morphogenesis of the crown serving merely to contain the stellate reticulum. It may, however, control the exchange of substances between the enamel organ and its environment. It is continuous with the inner enamel epithelium at the cervical loop where the two epithelia fold sharply upon each other to provide a stable rim to the enamel organ. Much later in time it will be seen that growth of the cervical loop provides the impetus for root formation. In early development the outer enamel epithelium is directly continuous, via the dental lamina, with the oral epithelium: the germ of the successional tooth will develop from its point of union with the lamina. Later the outer enamel epithelium is reinforced by the fibres of the dental follicle to assist in counteracting the internal pressures generated by the growing crown.

The mass of ectomesenchymal cells continues to increase in size but the steady encircling action of the enamel organ also continues until it surrounds such a large part of the dental papilla that the tooth germ takes on the appearance of a bell—the bell stage of tooth development (*Fig. 14F*). It is during this stage that the major cusps, ridges, and fissures of the ultimate crown pattern are established by the folding of the inner enamel epithelium. The dynamics of the folding process will form the subject of the next chapter and no more will be said at this stage.

At the early bell stage of development a new layer of cells differentiates within the enamel organ. This is the stratum intermedium. Presumably this layer is derived from the cells inside the enamel organ, perhaps from the diminishing enamel knot. It has been suggested that cells from this new layer may insinuate between the now columnar cells of the inner enamel epithelium helping to increase the surface area of this encircling layer.

During development each tooth germ is surrounded by a follicle or sac derived from ectomesenchymal cells displaced outwards from the presumptive dental papilla by the growing margin of the cervical loop. Beneath the tooth germ the follicle is continuous with the deep surface of the dental papilla, the vessels and nerves supplying the latter passing through it.

Within the follicle the developing tooth is able to undergo slight positional adjustments caused by growth forces generated during crown development. At the same time the follicle provides sufficient reinforcement to prevent the distortion of the outer enamel epithelium by forces from within the tooth germ. Though some of the follicle is destroyed when the tooth erupts, it will be seen in a later chapter that this tissue forms the basis of the periodontal ligament which maintains the functional tooth in its bony socket.

The application of highly sophisticated experimental techniques to very early developmental stages of amphibia have shown that the early embryo is differentiated into a mosaic of 'organization fields', each making a specific contribution to the definitive animal under the influence of chemical substances called 'evocators'.

In general terms, an anteroposterior (head–tail) polarity is established at an early stage in the developing embryo. The anterior pole is more advanced and from here a gradient of differentiation diminishes towards the posterior region. Within this major gradient further minor gradients develop. The major gradient results in (for instance) the successive differentiation of vertebrae which are probably all built up under the control of the same genetic influence; bodies, pedicles, laminae, and transverse processes are common to all but there is a gradual variation between successive vertebrae. Such a series is known as a 'meristic' series. The dentition may be another meristic series built from a minor gradient. Each tooth is based on a common plan of root, crown, and pulp chamber. Each quadrant of the mammalian dentition is thought to arise within a continuous morphogenetic field or gradient extending throughout the length of the jaw quadrant. Within this minor gradient there are fields of incisivation, caninization, and molarization such that according to which of these morphogenetic influences acts upon it, the undifferentiated tooth germ produces one or other of these tooth forms (*Fig. 16*).

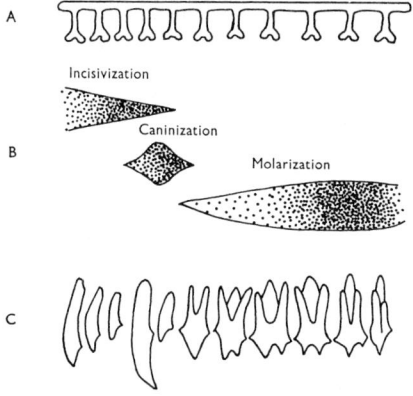

Fig. 16.—Diagrammatic representation of hypothetical differentiation of the mammalian dentition. A, The dental lamina with undifferentiated tooth germs; B, Morphogenetic fields believed to influence the development of the tooth germs; C, The resulting definitive dentition. (*Reproduced from Butler*, 1939.)

It will be observed that although there is some overlapping of the fields each has its own locus of maximum effect. In the human dentition the first permanent molar is most greatly influenced by the molarization field, the second and third molars to a lesser degree. This hypothesis provides a feasible step in the explanation of such phenomena as, for example, the molarization of the premolars in the dentition of the horse. It suggests that in this animal the molarization field extends as far forwards as the caninization field which is, however, poorly developed. However, it must be stated that there is no evidence to support this theory; it is merely a useful concept.

A further concept (also lacking experimental support) proposes that embryonic jaws of mammals contain three major developmental segments: incisor, canine and molar segments. During their evolution these segments have been able to expand either anteriorly or posteriorly but, in eutherian mammals, the incisor segment spreads back to produce the deciduous incisors in anteroposterior sequences; the canine region no longer spreads and therefore generates a single tooth; the molar region spreads anteriorly to generate the deciduous molars in sequence from back to front, and posteriorly to generate the permanent molars from front to back. The above three regions are each genetically coded for a different tooth pattern. The shape and size of a tooth depends on its position in a 'budding' sequence (*Fig. 17*). For example, in most eutherian mammals, the deciduous molars are initiated in sequence from the back to the front of the jaws. It is suggested that this sequence in which tooth buds are initiated determines the corresponding sequential decrease in the complexity of the deciduous molars and their

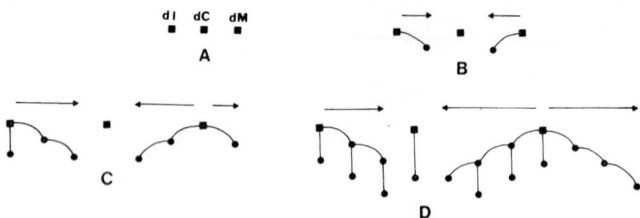

Fig. 17.—The jaws of eutherian mammals are supposed to contain 3 developmental segments; incisor, canine, and molar (D). The teeth in each segment are budded in sequence from 3 'stem' tooth families (A). These sequences (A–D) determine the gradients in tooth shape. Squares represent the 'stem' tooth buds; circles represent teeth; vertical lines connect deciduous teeth with their replacements; the arcs connect deciduous teeth of the same segment.

successors, the premolars (*Fig. 17*). However, it should be pointed out that in some mammals, including primates, it appears that the penultimate deciduous molar (e.g. the first deciduous molar in man) is the first postcanine to be initiated.

In this chapter we have discussed some aspects of the developmental processes affecting the tooth germ through its early stages up to the establishment of its 'bell' form. The next chapter will deal with the morphogenetic processes leading to the generation of the crown topography.

REFERENCES

De Beer G. R. (1947) The differentiation of neural crest cells into visceral cartilages and odontoblasts in ambystoma, and a re-examination of the germ-layer theory. *Proc. R. Soc.* **134-B,** 377.
Butler P. M. (1939) 1, Studies of the mammalian dentition. Differentiation of the post-canine dentition. *Proc. Zool. Soc. Lond.* **109-B,** 1.

Butler P. M. (1967) Dental merism and tooth development. *J. Dent. Res.* **46,** 845.

Fitzgerald L. R. (1969) Mechanisms controlling morphogenesis in developing teeth. *J. Dent. Res.* **48,** 726.

Gaunt W. A. and Miles A. E. W. (1967) Fundamental aspects of tooth morphogenesis. In: Miles A. E. W. (ed.), *Structural and Chemical Organization of Teeth* vol. 1. New York, Academic.

Ooe, T. (1957) On the early development of human dental lamina. *Okajimas Folia Anat. Jap.* **30,** 197.

Osborn J. W. (1973) The evolution of dentitions. *Am. Scient.* **61,** 548.

Pourtos M. (1961) 'Contribution a l'étude des bourgeons dentaires chez la souris. 1, Periodes d'induction et de morphodifferentiation', *Archs Biol. Liège* **72,** 17.

Scott J. H. (1967) *Dento-facial Growth and Development.* London, Pergamon.

Scott J. H. and Symons N. B. B. (1964) *Introduction to Dental Anatomy.* London, Livingstone.

Sicher H. (1962) *Orban's Oral Histology and Embryology.* St. Louis, Mosby.

Tonge C. H. (1953) The early development of teeth. *Proc. R. Soc. Med.* **46,** 313.

CHAPTER 6

THE DETERMINATION OF CROWN PATTERN

A MAJOR problem in developmental biology poses the question, 'How is shape developed?' We know that the shape of a protein is determined by its sequence of amino-acids and that this sequence is represented by a corresponding sequence of nucleic acids (DNA). But practically nothing is known of how the shapes of larger structures (for example, ameloblasts, fibroblasts, feathers, claws, fingers, hands, arms, or a cat) are controlled. To state that these shapes are genetically determined provides little advance on a theory of divine creation. Therefore, in order to understand how shape is generated we need to know what are the relevant cellular forces and how they are controlled; and little or nothing is known about either. The tooth could be one of the best experimental models for investigating this major problem.

All human lower right first molars look alike and are quite different from those of a cat. The many similarities between the teeth of animals comprising each mammalian species and their differences from the teeth of other mammalian species make it quite obvious that the occlusal morphology of a tooth is to a great extent genetically determined. From a detailed study of molar morphology in identical human twins it has been suggested that the presence and shape of even quite minor cuspules and fissures are probably genetically determined. Were it not for this study it might have been argued that local mechanical differences accounted for all minor variations between teeth. Similar studies have shown that the shape of the shovel-shaped incisor is also genetically determined. But these genetic studies do not reveal the mechanisms operating on the ball of cells comprising a tooth bud inducing it to develop its own unique shape.

The most obvious and consistent differences between the different teeth of the human dentition are their size, occlusal morphology, and the distribution and number of roots. In this chapter we will consider what is known about the way in which the characteristic occlusal morphology of a tooth is developed.

At the cap stage of tooth development there are obvious differences between the sizes of different tooth germs. These differences can presumably be related to either a more rapid or a longer lasting phase of cell division in the larger tooth germs. However, it is only in the bell stage that distinct morphological differences between

38

tooth germs can be recognized. In the previous chapter a concept was discussed which suggests that these differences are brought about under the influence of tooth fields.

This theory has been investigated in the following way. At a critical stage in the embryonic development of mouse teeth the oral epithelium in a jaw quadrant was carefully separated from the underlying mesenchyme and replaced in such a way that the molar epithelium covered the incisor region and the incisor epithelium covered the molar region. The jaw quadrant was now cultured *in vitro*. For a short while the teeth continued to develop in the culture medium. Subsequently these teeth rudiments were studied and it appeared that molariform teeth were developing in the incisor region and incisiform teeth were developing in the molar region. This particular study and other studies on amphibia suggest that different regions of the oral epithelium (rather than the underlying ectomesenchyme) are initially responsible for determining the different occlusal morphologies of teeth.

However, a different series of experiments leads to the opposite conclusion. Incisor and molar buds were dissected from the jaws of embryo mice at a rather later stage of development than that used in the previous study. The ectodermal and ectomesenchymal parts of the buds were separated: the incisor ectoderm was grafted onto the molar ectomesenchyme and the molar ectoderm onto the incisor ectomesenchyme. Organ culture of the recombinations revealed that the shape of the resultant tooth was determined by the ectomesenchyme. The ectomesenchyme also possessed the ability to control the activity of embryonic ectoderm from many other sites. For example, ectoderm which would have developed into epithelium covering the foot, or into hair follicles, was induced by a molar dental papilla to grow into the enamel organ of a molar tooth. These experiments suggest that the ectomesenchyme of a tooth bud determines the shape into which a tooth develops (*see also* Chapter 5).

Neither of the above experiments reveal whether morphogenetic fields (Chapter 5) exist or whether the shape into which a tooth develops is determined by its position in a 'budding sequence'.

It is during the bell stage of tooth development that the ultimate occlusal morphologies of teeth begin to be established in such a way that it is possible to recognize differences between those germs which will develop into incisor, canine, premolar and molar teeth. The following theory attempts to explain on a mechanistic basis some of the forces which may be generated within the tooth germ and which may bring about these differences.

The occlusal morphology of a tooth is the outcome of two features. The first is the shape of the enamel-dentine junction. But this shape is not exactly the same as that of the occlusal surface of the tooth.

Minor variations, particularly in the form of small cuspules and fissures, are produced due to regional variations in the thickness of the enamel deposited on the enamel-dentine junction. Apart from documenting their existence no study of the development of these minor variations in enamel thickness appears to have been made, although it seems possible that the constriction of the blood-supply to ameloblasts in the region of fissures is related to the thin enamel which may be found in these regions. The theory referred to above discusses the way in which the internal enamel epithelium folds to establish the shape of the presumptive enamel-dentine junction. It is only when the first layers of enamel and dentine have been deposited on either side of this junction that its definitive shape is established.

The developing tooth germ may be likened to a fluid-filled sphere which is partitioned across the middle by the inner enamel epithelium. The stellate reticulum is on one side of the partition and the dental papilla on the other side (*Fig. 18A*). The cells of the stellate

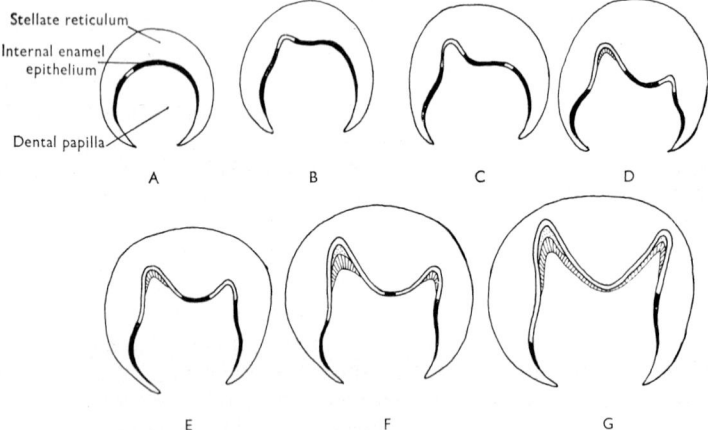

Fig. 18.—Seven stages in the folding of the internal enamel epithelium. Regions in which the cells of the internal enamel epithelium are dividing are black; regions in which division has ceased are clear. Enamel is stippled, dentine is cross-hatched. Cusps continue to separate while the cells of the internal enamel epithelium are dividing. The final shape of the enamel-dentine junction is stabilized when the dentine bridge has connected the two cusps (G).

reticulum are separated from each other by acidic mucopolysaccharide. This substance is intensely hydrophilic and the water which it has absorbed is thought to produce a region of high hydrostatic pressure. On the other side of the partition the growing dental papilla balances this hydrostatic pressure so that the internal enamel epithelium is stabilized between the two. The surrounding dental follicle constricts the tooth germ to an approximately spherical shape. The partitioning sheet of cells (the internal enamel epithelium) increases in surface area by cell division. But its perimeter, the cervical loop, is prevented from expanding by the retaining dental follicle. Evidently, as the surface area of the partition increases it must buckle. By this buckling a primary cuspal elevation of the internal enamel epithelium is produced (*Fig. 18B*). From a purely mechanistic analogy it might be thought that the internal enamel epithelium could buckle down into the dental papilla rather than up into the stellate reticulum. But it will be remembered that the surface of the dental papilla is convex towards the internal enamel epithelium and this will result in any mechanical buckling being towards the stellate reticulum.

It has been observed that mitotic activity has now ceased in the region of the cuspal elevation of the internal enamel epithelium and that adjacent odontoblasts rapidly become differentiated and dentine is soon deposited. However, cell division continues in the internal enamel epithelium flanking the primary cuspal elevation. These flanks are now convex towards the dental papilla so that from a purely mechanistic analogy it can be argued that the growing internal enamel epithelium would now begin to buckle into the dental papilla. This does in fact occur so that the height of the primary cuspal elevation is increased by a deepening of its flanks down into the dental papilla rather than further growth up into the stellate reticulum (*Fig. 18B*).

At this stage, if another cusp is to be formed, cell division of the internal enamel epithelium ceases in the region which will correspond with this secondary cusp. Just as in the formation of the primary cusp, so a secondary cuspal elevation develops on the flanks of the now mineralizing primary cusp (*Fig. 18C*). This region becomes rapidly stabilized by the differentiation of odontoblasts and the laying down of dentine. Meanwhile cell division between the two cusps continues so that the internal enamel epithelium buckles further into the papilla thus increasing both the heights and the separation between the now mineralizing cusps (*Fig. 18E–G*).

To summarize, it appears that cell division of the sheet of internal enamel epithelium first ceases in the region of what will be the primary cusp of the tooth (*Fig. 19*). This is followed by a buckling of the internal enamel epithelium in this region, the differentiation of odontoblasts, and the laying down of dentine. If further cusps are to be formed cell division in the internal enamel epithelium ceases at the tips of these presumptive secondary cusps which are situated down the flanks of the primary cuspal elevation. The sequence of development of the cusps in equivalent multi-cusped teeth is usually the same.

41

The experiments referred to above suggest that, by the time a tooth bud has been formed, the dental papilla controls tooth shape, presumably by controlling mitotic activity in the adjacent internal enamel epithelium. But how does it determine the sites at which the internal enamel epithelium ceases to divide and initiate the differentiation of presumptive ameloblasts?

Recent work suggests that cAMP (cyclic adenine monophosphate) and cGMP (cyclic guanine monophosphate) may be involved. A very small proportion of the ATP in cells may be broken down by an intracellular enzyme into cAMP. The amount is infinitesimal

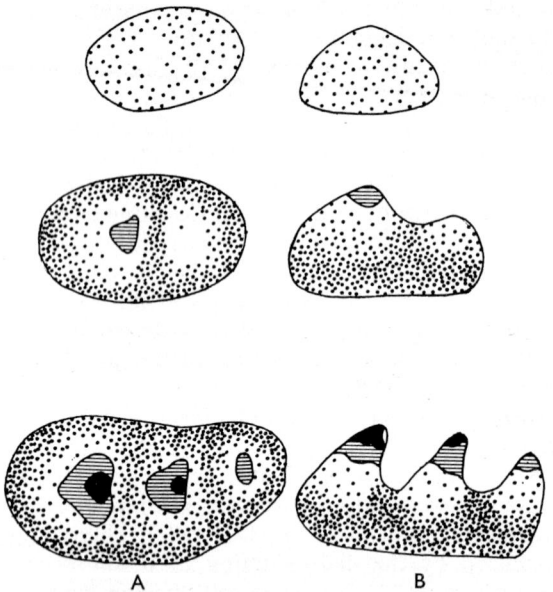

Fig. 19.—Diagram representing the distribution of dividing cells in the inner dental epithelium of a mouse molar at three successive developmental stages. A, In occlusal view; B, In side view. Not to scale. Solid black area represents forming enamel, lined area forming dentine. Each dot signifies a dividing cell.

because about 1 000 kg of body tissue may be required to produce 10 μg of cAMP: however, the substance can be synthesized *in vitro* and its activity inhibited *in vivo* in order to facilitate studies of its function(s). It appears that cAMP induces the differentiation of cells while cGMP induces cell division and growth. It might therefore be supposed that during growth of the tooth germ the cells of the papilla produce cGMP which is passed into the basement membrane between the dental papilla and the internal enamel epithelium. In this position it may become attached to the plasma

42

membranes of the internal enamel epithelium, and in some way initiate cell division. At a later stage the papilla cells will produce less cGMP and more cAMP. This latter substance inhibits cell division and encourages the differentiation of ameloblasts.

The above speculations, even if correct, still leave a crucial question unanswered: if the dental papilla controls tooth shape, how does it control the positions at which the internal enamel epithelium stops dividing? If a rabbit molar germ is bisected, each half develops into a molar. This seems to suggest that the feature which organizes the shape of the tooth is represented in each half of the dental papilla, and perhaps in every ectomesenchymal cell of the papilla.

The cusps of teeth are not the smooth symmetrical cones which would be expected to develop from the simple mechanical explanation given above. Even the human canine possesses ridges running from near the cusp tip to the cervical margin of the crown, while close inspection of unworn molars reveals a variety of ridges associated with each cusp, apparently having little or no functional or phylogenetic significance. While many of these features may be accounted for by localized enamel thickenings, those of a more permanent nature, e.g. the oblique ridges of human upper molars, are established at the enamel dentine junction. Investigation into the distribution of dividing cells in developing molars reveals that growth is not even over the entire surface. Indeed, there is often a greater proportion of dividing cells of the inner enamel epithelium over one flank of a cusp than another, so that it can be argued that tensional forces are set up which cause the cusp to tilt slightly on the crown. This has been shown in the carnassial teeth of the cat. Until mineralization starts the crown pattern remains pliable and ridges can form, to be stabilized later by the formation of hard dentine and enamel along their crests: there is evidence that apposition of enamel spreads more rapidly along the ridges than over the intervening cuspal surfaces. The ridges so formed serve not only to link the cusps and produce a characteristic crown pattern, but also to provide functional shearing edges. Moreover, the complex of ridges tends to generate intervening fossae into which cusps of the opposing teeth can bite to provide a pestle-and-mortar action.

In the above paragraph it was mentioned that until it has been stabilized by the development of mineralized tissues, the crown pattern can be deformed. Thus, if it were possible temporarily to inhibit dentine development, the internal enamel epithelium might be deformed into a different shape. Based on reconstructions of human tooth germs at different stages of development, it has been suggested that the different shapes and sizes of the first and second deciduous molars and the first permanent molar may be related to a progressive delay in the onset of the formation of dentine in the later developed teeth.

So far little mention has been made regarding the role of the dental papilla in determining the crown pattern. Without the papilla no dentine would form, hence the folds of the inner enamel epithelium would not be stabilized. In fact, early in development the crown pattern is formed in dentine which serves to provide the template over which enamel is later deposited (*Fig. 18G*). In the early stages of development mitosis figures can be observed in the peripheral papilla cells, although the exact correspondence with those in the inner dental epithelium claimed by some does not occur. The papilla follows faithfully the profile of the inner enamel epithelium and may restrain any tendency of the epithelium towards excessive folding. As will become apparent in later chapters, the inner enamel epithelium obtains its nutriment via the papilla until the formation of dentine separates it from this source. Thus the papilla has a nutritive role, at least up to the time of dentine formation. Though there is as yet no direct evidence, it has been argued that growth centres located in the papilla are responsible for controlling the growth in outline of the base of the crown, hence the size of the tooth and incidentally the number and disposition of the roots. Unquestionably the ectodermal and ectomesenchymal components of the tooth germ must work in close co-ordination to produce the topographical pattern of a crown. However, the present state of our knowledge does not allow us to say whether small teeth arise from a small number of initial cells.

It would appear, then, that while the definitive tooth results from developmental interaction between the enamel organ and the dental papilla, the intrinsic growth of the inner enamel epithelium causes this layer to fold in a predetermined manner, so as to generate a genetically reproducible pattern of cusps, ridges, and fissures which become stabilized by the dentine and enamel. In the following chapter we shall review the evidence concerning the role of the soft tissue components of the tooth germ in the context of tooth growth.

REFERENCES

Butler P. M. (1956) The ontogeny of molar pattern. *Biol. Rev.* **31**, 30.

Dryburg L. C. (1967) The epigenetics of early tooth development in the mouse. *J. Dent. Res.* **46**, 1264.

Gaunt W. A. (1955) The development of the molar pattern of the mouse. *Acta Anat.* **24**, 249.

Gaunt W. A. (1959) The development of the deciduous cheek teeth of the cat. *Acta Anat.* **38**, 187.

Gaunt W. A. (1961a) The presence of apical pits on the lower cheek teeth of the mouse. *Acta Anat.* **44**, 146.

Gaunt W. A. (1961b) The development of the molar pattern of the golden hamster. *Acta Anat.* **45,** 219.

Gaunt W. A. and Miles A. E. W. (1967) *See* Chapter 5.

Kraus B. S. and Jordan R. E. (1965) *The Human Dentition before Birth.* London, Kimpton.

Miller W. A. (1969) Inductive changes in early tooth development: 1, A study of mouse tooth development on the chick chorioallantois. *J. Dent. Res.* **48,** 719.

Slavkin H. C. and Bavetta L. A. (1972) *Developmental Aspects of Oral Biology.* New York, Academic.

Wood B. F. and Green L. J. (1968) Second premolar morphologic trait similarities in twins. *J. Dent. Res.* **48,** 74.

CHAPTER 7

GROWTH OF THE TOOTH GERM

THE term 'growth' encompasses all the processes involving increase in size and weight of the individual from the time of fertilization of the egg. In the two preceding chapters some of the histological changes within the tooth germ from its time of inception have been indicated but little has so far been said concerning the progressive changes in the dimensions of the developing tooth germ. In this dimensional sense growth involves changes not only in absolute size but also in the relative proportions of the component parts, both of which determine the definitive form.

Before proceeding further it will be helpful to mention briefly some of the techniques available for measuring growth of tooth germs. It is possible by careful microdissection to free the developing tooth germs from the surrounding tissues and to measure their gross dimensions directly. However, owing to the amount of fluid in the stellate reticulum and the delicate nature of the outer enamel epithelium in the early tooth germ, great care is necessary to prevent the enamel organ collapsing and causing distortion of the inner enamel epithelium. With the onset of dentinogenesis, the dentine caps can be dissected out and stained with alizarin red S which differentially stains mineralized regions on the tooth crown. Alternatively, whole jaws may be stained with alizarin red solution and then rendered transparent to allow direct measurements of the stained dentine caps *in situ*. The total volumes of enamel and dentine formed can be measured directly from dissected teeth. When mineralized, the dentine and enamel caps become radio-opaque and their dimensions can be measured directly by radiographs *in vivo*.

However, from the two previous chapters it is clear that much of the crown pattern is defined by the soft tissues before mineralization starts, and that the crown form results from developmental interaction between the enamel organ and the dental papilla, neither of whose dimensions can be measured accurately except in histological sections. Therefore, in order to study the growth of the very early germ, and especially the relative contribution of the soft tissue components, serial sections of histologically fixed tooth germs have been laboriously analysed. Each technique is suited to investigating a particular developmental stage of the tooth germ, the collected results depicting the overall growth picture.

46

From what has already been said concerning cusp development it is clear that the distances between developing cusp tips increase as the crown becomes larger (*Fig. 18D–F*). It will be recalled that the cusps sometimes tilt during development and this is an additional factor determining intercuspal distance. Once the spreading front of mineralized tissue reaches the floors of the intervening valleys, the flanking dentine cusps are stabilized and their intercuspal distances remain constant (*Fig. 18G*). Any further changes in the sharpness of ridges and cusps will then be due to differences in the thickness of enamel secreted on the dentine template.

Consider the two ways in which the length of the internal enamel epithelium might increase during development. During the cap stage, all these epithelial cells seem to be capable of dividing and no ameloblasts are being differentiated. This suggests that there would be a continuous increase in the number of dividing cells and therefore that growth would accelerate. But at a later stage growth is confined to the cervical loop, and it might be that for each cell which now divides another differentiates to become an ameloblast. Under these conditions the number of dividing cells would remain constant and growth would be constant rather than accelerating. We could distinguish between these two types of growth by measuring the length of the internal enamel epithelium in tooth germs of different ages. If growth is constant, and length is plotted against age, the resultant line would be straight, but if growth accelerates the line would be curved. For the latter case, ideal conditions would lead to a straight line if log length were plotted against time.

Most growth studies reveal an initial acceleration from a slow start, followed by a constant rate of increase ending with a period of deceleration. Consider growth in the mesiodistal diameter of human lower first deciduous molars (*Fig. 20*). We can distinguish two parts of this curve; it is straight up till about 22 weeks and then it is curved. Because length (mesiodistal diameter) rather than log length has been plotted against time, we might conclude that from 11 to 22 weeks the number of dividing cells does not significantly increase. In other words, many of the dividing cells are differentiating rather than contributing to an increase in the population of dividing cells.

When both cusps start to mineralize the rate of growth decreases, and when they are joined by dentine across the middle of the tooth (starred in *Fig. 20*) the decrease in growth rate becomes more obvious. The apparent absence of an initial acceleration in the growth rate demonstrated by *Fig. 20* is probably due to the fact that data for all 11-day tooth germs have been pooled. Thus, the measurement at this time (about 0·8 mm) includes tooth germs which

47

may range from 0·2 to 1·2 mm (for instance). It is probably during increase from 0·1 mm to 1·2 mm that growth is accelerating.

It has been shown for lower deciduous molars that the rate of growth in the mesiodistal diameter exceeds that in the buccolingual diameter (*Fig. 21*). Hence the definitive crown is longer than it is

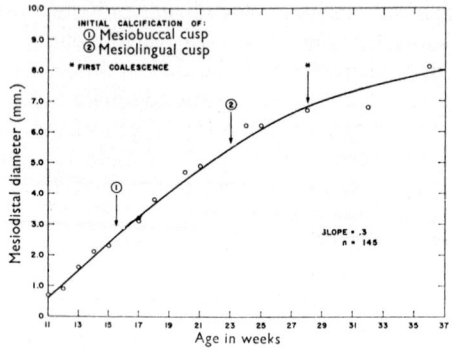

Fig. 20.—Graph of mean mesiodistal diameters of mandibular first primary molars plotted against age. (*Figs. 20–22 reproduced from Kraus and Jordan, 1965.*)

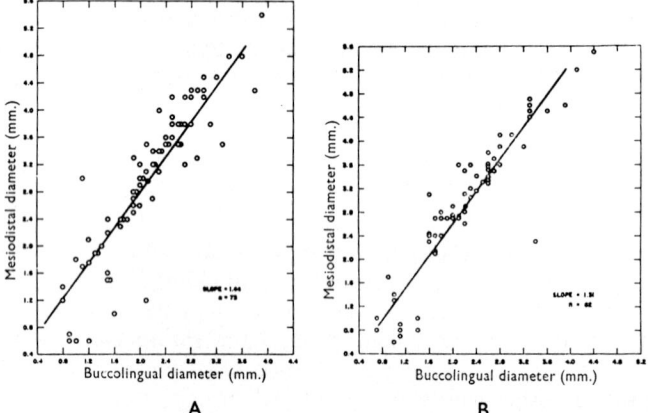

A   B

Fig. 21.—Graphs of mesiodistal diameters of, **A**, mandibular first primary molars and, **B**, mandibular second primary molars, plotted against buccolingual diameters.

broad. The corresponding upper primary molars grow more rapidly along the buccolingual than the mediodistal diameter and the result-ant crown is broader than long (*Fig. 22*). Similar results have been obtained from measurements of developing mouse molars. These teeth all grow very rapidly by increase in size and number of cells up to the time of completion of the crown pattern which roughly coincides with the appearance of the mineralized tissues. Thereafter, a slower rate of growth continues by accretion of enamel.

Consider, now, growth in height of the tooth. The height of the enamel organ measured along an axis passing vertically through its

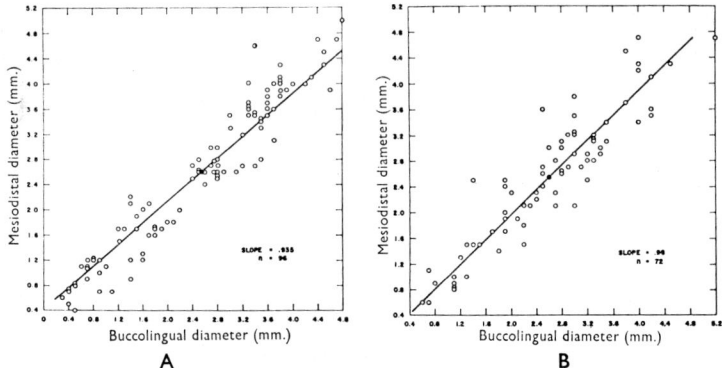

Fig. 22.—Graphs of mesiodistal diameters of, A, maxillary first primary molars and, B, maxillary second primary molars, plotted against buccolingual diameters.

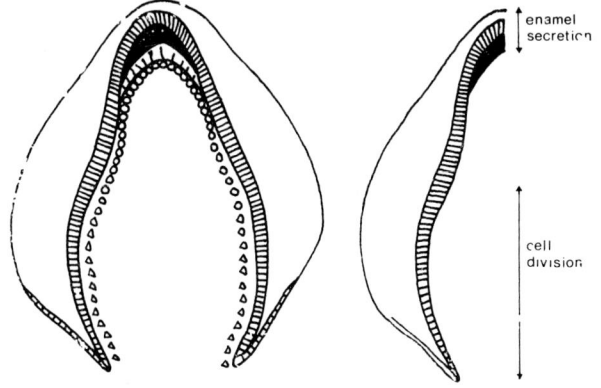

Fig. 23.—The crown height of a growing tooth is contributed by enamel and by the internal enamel epithelium.

centre is contributed by the internal enamel epithelium, some of whose cells are dividing and some of which have ceased dividing, and by the cuspal enamel together with its associated enamel organ (*Fig. 23*). The height of the tooth can be increased by the deposition of cuspal enamel or by an increase in the height of the internal

49

enamel epithelium (at the cervical loop) due to cell division. Enamel is deposited at the same rate in most human teeth (about 4 μm/day). Therefore *differences* in the rates at which teeth grow in height must be due to *differences* in the rate at which the internal enamel epithelium grows in height. This will depend on two factors; the time it takes each cell to divide and the size of the population of dividing cells. It is differences in this latter population which probably account for differences in the rates at which the heights of teeth increase. The size of this population depends on the rate of cell division, and on the rate at which cells are removed from this population by differentiating into ameloblasts (which do not divide). Therefore, if the rate of cell differentiation is slowed down, we might expect the height of the tooth to increase more rapidly because more and more dividing cells are being produced. From measurements of growing deciduous molars and first permanent molars it appears that the increased height of first molars is due to a delay in the times at which cells differentiate.

It is known that the tissue components of the developing mouse molar do not all grow at the same rate. The rate of growth of the surface area of the inner enamel epithelium is most rapid up to the time of completion of the definitive shape of the presumptive enamel-dentine junction. During this time, mitosis figures are abundant in the inner dental epithelium particularly in the presumptive cingulum zone, and growth consists essentially of cell multiplication. This is the time when the inner enamel epithelium is functioning as a surface of metabolic exchange between the enamel organ and the papilla and coincides with a maximum vascular supply to the papilla. Although little corresponding evidence is yet available for the human developing tooth, occasional references are encountered in the literature showing a similar pattern of distribution of mitosis figures, so that it is reasonable to suppose the growth processes in the different teeth to be closely comparable (*Fig. 24*). In the mouse molars the enamel organ has a slightly greater volume than the dental papilla up to the time of crown pattern completion, though both components grow at the same rate. Later, however, as the stellate reticulum becomes reduced, the enamel organ shrinks, becoming smaller than the dental papilla. Descriptive accounts, as opposed to actual measurements, suggest that the enamel organ grows rapidly in a basal direction to enshroud the papilla, but in the mouse at least it is known that this apparent enshrouding is in reality due to an overall change in shape of the inner enamel epithelium from hemispherical to conical.

This suggests that descriptive accounts of developing human teeth need to be checked by actual measurements of the component tissues of the dental organ.

In general terms, then, the present state of our knowledge enables us to say that growth of the tooth germ comprises two phases. During the first (soft tissue) phase the dental organ rapidly changes in both size and shape. Cells are rapidly dividing and morphogenetic

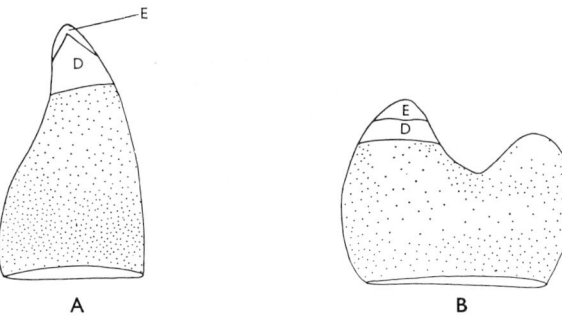

A   B

Fig. 24.—Distribution of dividing cells in the inner dental epithelium of human tooth germs. A, |B. Note the greater density of dividing cells in the cingulum zone. B, D|. Note area of dividing cells between the cusps. Not to scale. D, dentine; E, enamel.

processes are taking place. In the succeeding (hard tissue) phase the shape has already been established and there is only growth in size due to the deposition of enamel and dentine. The rate of cell division is waning and hard tissues are being deposited.

REFERENCES

Butler P. M. (1968) Growth of the human second lower deciduous molar. *Archs Oral Biol.* **13,** 671.

Butler P. M. (1971) In: Dahlberg A. A. (ed.), *Dental Morphology and Evolution.* Chicago, University of Chicago Press, p. 3.

Christensen G. J. (1967) Occlusal morphology of human molar tooth buds. *Archs Oral Biol.* **12,** 141.

Gaunt W. A. (1963) An analysis of the growth of the cheek teeth of the mouse. *Acta Anat.* **54,** 220.

Kraus B. S. and Jordan R. E. (1965). *See* Chapter 6.

Stack M. V. (1964) A gravimetric study of crown growth rate of the human deciduous dentition. *Biol. Neonat.* **6,** 197.

Turner E. P. (1963) Crown development in human deciduous molar teeth. *Archs Oral Biol.* **8,** 523.

CHAPTER 8

THE BLOOD SUPPLY TO THE TEETH

IN studying the vascular supply to the dental tissues, it is necessary to determine the origin of the vessels, their arrangement, distribution, and density both within and around the tooth. Where tissue development is rapid there is a rich blood supply, and the more complex the organization of the particular structure, whether anatomically or physiologically, the more abundant are the anastomoses of blood capillaries to be found. Density of the capillary network is most important in controlling the growth of the tissue, for on it depends the hypertrophy or atrophy of the tissue supplied. Abnormal blood supply leads to hypertrophy or atrophy of the whole or parts of the tooth, irregularities of surface configuration, defects in quality of the organic or inorganic components, and other structural or physiological deviations from the typical form.

Although it is possible by laborious analysis of serial sections to reconstruct a panoramic view of vascular distribution to the teeth, the majority of investigations so far reported are based upon procedures involving the replacement of the blood in the vessels by an injected mass whose properties determine the techniques of examination subsequently employed. Coloured dyes, india ink, tinted latex, or coloured precipitates formed within the vessels by interaction between injected chemicals, all reveal the vascular architecture with great clarity, especially when combined with bulk clearing the whole specimens, rendering them transparent. In recent years acid corrosion techniques have been developed. The surrounding tissues are removed by a corrosive fluid, leaving a three-dimensional model of the vascular system. Radio-opaque injection media enable the vascular pattern to be studied radiographically. Two new techniques have recently proved useful in studies of vascular distribution. One technique involves the use of plastic microspheres of known dimension which are injected directly into an artery and allowed to circulate. The microspheres lodge in that portion of the vascular bed where the vessels are of the same diameter as the microspheres. When histological sections are examined the plastic microspheres are clearly seen marking the vessels in which they have lodged. In this way the distribution of any selected part of the arterial system can be studied. The second technique is the histochemical demonstration of adenosine tri-phosphatase (ATP-ase) in blood vessel walls.

Two basic difficulties are common to all injection techniques. First, the substance must be injected into fresh material under sufficient pressure to fill completely the vascular system but not so great as to rupture the vessels. This gives a picture of the entire vascular bed. However, the entire vascular bed is not fully patent at any one time during life; the pressure applied at the time of injection must certainly have opened a proportion of the smaller channels which would normally be temporarily collapsed. The second problem arises from the technical difficulty of representing a three-dimensional system on a two-dimensional picture. Though absence of the third dimension in the illustrations can be compensated for by written description, the entire complexity of the injected system can only be seen in the original model.

The few published accounts concerning blood-supply to primate and human dentitions are in broad agreement with the much more detailed investigations relating to the corresponding system in small mammals. Hence, the picture of vascular supply to the teeth presented in the following paragraphs will be a composite one.

The mammalian upper teeth and their supporting tissues all derive their blood-supply from branches of the superior dental arteries, supplemented to varying degrees by branches of the palatal vessels. The corresponding lower teeth and their supporting structures are supplied by branches of the inferior dental arteries which lie within the inferior dental canals; additional supply is derived from branches of the lingual vessels. As stated in Chapter 4, these vessels are present in the jaws of very early cat embryos, even before the appearance of tooth germs. From these as yet thin-walled vessels capillaries arise which are concentrated along the jaws in localized regions which indicate the sites of future tooth germs. In the regions between the future tooth germs, and also in the rodent diastema, there is a sharp reduction in the capillary concentration. Such vascular arrangements have not been reported in primate or human fetal jaws, though it is very probable that here too a closely comparable situation could be demonstrated.

Reconstructions of mammalian and primate tooth germs from serial sections show that groups of blood vessels, originating from the superior and inferior dental arteries, first pass into the dental papilla at the cap stage of development. Detailed analysis of these vessels in the mouse molars (*Fig. 25*) shows that they increase in number during the period of histo-differentiation of the tooth germ, reaching a maximum concentration immediately before the phase of most active folding of the inner dental epithelium. Gradually, with the onset of dentinogenesis, the number of vessels decreases and then becomes stabilized for that particular tooth. It will also be seen from *Fig. 25* that the total blood flow, computed from the mean

53

diameters of the vessels, increases in parallel manner during this vital morphogenetic period.

At no time during development do blood vessels penetrate into the enamel organ, so that up to the start of dentinogenesis the inner enamel epithelium probably obtains the majority of its nutrient via the papillary vessels rather than via the outer enamel epithelium.

It would thus appear that when dentine is produced it forms a barrier which prevents further metabolic exchange between the enamel organ and the dental papilla. This suggestion has received

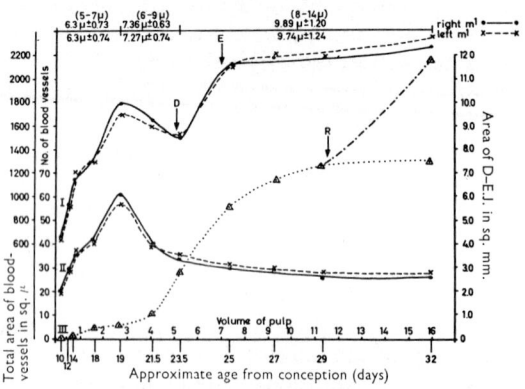

Fig. 25.—Graphs showing: I, the total cross-sectional area of blood-vessels entering the base of the dental papilla in the upper first mouse molar; II, the numbers of such vessels; and, III, the area of the enamel-dentine junction, all plotted against age. D, Time of start of dentinogenesis; E, time of start of amelogenesis; R, onset of root formation. The mean diameters of the vessels are shown. (*Figs. 25 and 26 modified from Gaunt*, 1960.)

support from histochemical evidence and from the cytological re-arrangement of the organelles within the cells of the inner enamel epithelium (*see* Chapter 15). Lying adjacent to the outer enamel epithelium is a plexus of blood vessels which originate partly from the basal vessels before they pass into the dental papilla, and partly from the periosteal plexus associated with the developing tooth socket.

The blood vessels passing into the dental papilla branch succes-sively, their finest terminations pushing between the odontoblasts as capillary loops from a sub-odontoblastic plexus.

Before the roots are formed, the vessels entering the papilla congregate in groups whose number and position coincide with the number and location of the roots specific to that tooth (*Fig. 26*). It has been suggested that each of these vascular bundles supplies a separate growth centre within the papilla, though so far without conclusive evidence. As the tooth ages so the pulp chamber diminishes in volume (Chapter 23), the apical foramina become progressively narrowed by invading cement and the blood-supply becomes reduced. Thus it is that the tooth in old age receives but a very small proportion of its original blood-supply and the viability of the pulp diminishes.

The blood supply to the tissues surrounding the tooth which include the periodontal ligament, the gingiva, the alveolar bone, and the epithelial attachment must now be considered.

Examination of material, utilizing the techniques already described, reveals an astonishing vascular density in the tissues adjacent to the tooth. The main supply to the ligament is via the dental artery

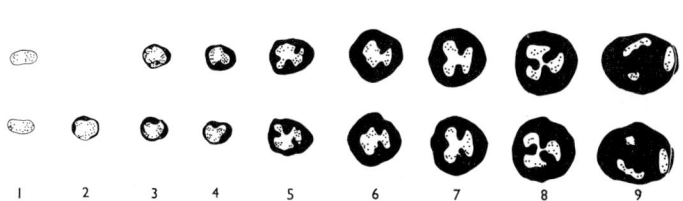

Fig. 26.—Apical views of the developing left and right second upper molar of the mouse showing the blood vessels entering the dental papilla. Each dot represents a blood vessel.

(*Fig. 27*). This artery initially has an intrabony course and gives off alveolar branches. One enters the periodontium apically, gives off two longitudinal periodontal arteries and then continues to supply the pulp. Interalveolar arteries ascend to the crest of the alveolus giving off many perforating branches which enter the periodontal ligament at right angles to the socket wall. At the crest of the alveolus these vessels continue on to supply the attachment epithelium and the col area. The perforating arteries are numerous and have been shown to increase in number from tooth to tooth towards the posterior teeth and, in single rooted teeth, to be greatest in number in the gingival third of the ligament and least in the middle third. The perforating arteries run parallel to the fibre bundles of the ligament and form an arcading network closer to the bone surface than to the cement surface. The classic description of longitudinal arteries running in the periodontal ligament has been questioned. When plastic microspheres are injected into the arterial system they are only found lodged in the perforating arteries. This means that either the longitudinal vessels described after injection techniques represent the venous return or are of such a diameter that the plastic microspheres do not lodge within their lumen. In view of the profuse

55

arterial supply via the socket wall it is more than likely that the longitudinal vessels are associated with the venous drainage of the ligament.

The blood supply to the gingiva and attachment apparatus shows distinct regional differences. The marginal and attached gingiva receive blood from vessels running in the periosteum of the alveolar process. Branches from these vessels run perpendicular to the surface and form loops within the connective tissue papillae of the gingiva. The vessels supplying the crevicular and attachment epithelium, however, show a different disposition. These are derived mainly

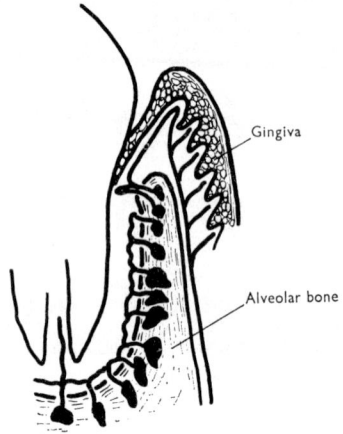

Gingiva

Alveolar bone

Fig. 27.—Diagram illustrating the arterial supply of the periodontium.

from intrabony arteries which leave the alveolar process in the crestal area and pursue a course close to and parallel with the epithelium forming a rich network of vessels. In the region of the col, vessels leave the crest of the alveolar bone, and run perpendicularly to the surface of the col. Close to the surface they bend sharply and run parallel to the basement membrane supporting the col epithelium. The difference in the spatial arrangement of vessels in the attached gingiva and the crevicular epithelium most likely reflects the differences in the architecture of the junction between epithelium and its supporting connective tissue. In the presence of inflammation the flat junction supporting the crevicular and attachment epithelium changes and pegs of proliferative epithelium are found. At the same time the vascular supply to this region now develops looped vessels.

Thus essentially the blood supply to the periodontium can be divided into three zones: that to the periodontal ligament, that to the gingiva facing the oral cavity, and that to the gingiva facing the tooth. However, anastomoses have been demonstrated between all three areas and this allows for a considerable collateral circulation in the supporting tissues of the tooth.

REFERENCES

Birn H. (1966) The vascular supply of the periodontal membrane. *J. Periodont. Res.* **1,** 51.

Egelberg J. (1966) The blood vessels of the dentino-gingival junction. *J. Periodont. Res.* **1,** 163.

Folke L. E. A. and Stallard R. E. (1967) Periodontal microcirculation as revealed by plastic microspheres. *J. Periodont. Res.* **2,** 53.

Gaunt W. A. (1960) The vascular supply in relation to the formation of roots on the cheek teeth of the mouse. *Acta Anat.* **43,** 116.

Kindlova M. (1965) The blood supply of the marginal periodontium in *Macacus rhesus. Archs Oral Biol.* **10,** 869.

CHAPTER 9

COLLAGEN

COLLAGEN is an essential constituent of connective tissues so that, apart from enamel, it is a component of all the dental tissues. As it has been suggested that collagen might be necessary for the initiation of mineralization, that it might provide the force for tooth eruption, and that it has a significant role to play in tooth support, it is obvious that some knowledge of this fibrous protein is necessary.

The chemical composition of collagen is unique. The amino-acids found in collagen fall into two obvious groups; those present in large amounts and those in small amounts. Two-thirds of the total amino-acids are represented by glycine, alanine, proline and hydroxyproline, whilst the remaining one-third consists of fourteen amino-acids. Two amino-acids found in collagen, hydroxyproline and hydroxylysine, are not generally found in other animal tissue proteins. The exceptions are complement and surfactant.

Collagen is synthesized by the fibroblast and although some steps in its synthesis are still unclear, the general outline of its formation has been established. Thus the individual amino-acids are assembled into polypeptide chains at the polysomes, each chain being coiled around its own axis in a simple left hand helix (*Fig. 28*). Incorporated within these chains are the amino-acids proline and lysine, which subsequently become hydroxylated before three such chains become linked together in a coiled right-handed helix like a three-stranded rope. This macromolecule is termed 'procollagen'. Each individual chain in the procollagen macromolecule is characterized by an amino-acid assemblage at its amino-terminal end which is clearly distinct from the rest of the chain. Before the procollagen macromolecule can be secreted by the fibroblast, these terminal groupings need to be removed and this is achieved by the action of an enzyme, procollagen peptidase. Once removed the 'collagen macromolecule', as it is now termed, is secreted. Outside the cell the collagen macromolecules then undergo aggregation with other collagen macromolecules to form collagen fibrils. The pathway of these events within the fibroblast is not certain. Autoradiographic studies using tritiated proline suggest a pathway from the polysomes to the Golgi apparatus via the endoplasmic reticulum: then from the Golgi apparatus to the cell surface in vesicles which eventually fuse with the cell membrane and release their contents. Unfortunately proline is not found exclusively in collagen, so its presence may demonstrate the synthesis by the fibroblast of some other material apart from collagen. Therefore procollagen may pass direct from the polysome to the cell surface. Very recently it has been established that in some cells the odontoblast and osteoblast (and most likely the fibroblast), the pathway of collagen synthesis, does involve the Golgi apparatus.

The mechanism whereby the collagen macromolecules are aggregated together is not certain but it probably first involves electrostatic forces between charged groups of neighbouring macromolecules. The evidence for this is as follows. Normal collagen fibrils when viewed with the electron microscope show a characteristic band repeating at every 64 nm. If a solution of collagen macromolecules is reconstituted in 1 per cent sodium chloride a fibril with a band repeating at 64 nm is formed. If the concentration of the electrolyte is varied collagen fibrils with a repeating band every 280 nm are produced. This effect of the electrolyte environment on the aggregation of collagen macromolecules is consistent with the presence of electrostatic forces between macromolecules. Thus in young collagen first formed after aggregation of the macromolecules there exists a triple helix of polypeptide chains joined together by hydrogen bonds which in turn are aggregated with similar units by means of electrostatic bonds. This is an extremely unstable state and probably only exists at the initial formation of the collagen fibrils, for it is known that collagen becomes progressively more stable and insoluble as collagen matures. Collagen maturation involves the formation of additional strong cross-linkages in the form of covalent bonds. These cross-linkages occur between the individual polypeptide chains and also between the collagen macromolecules.

The way in which the collagen macromolecules aggregate to give the structural basis of collagen with its characteristic 64 nm banding as seen with the electron microscope is not certain. It has been suggested that each macromolecule has five bonding zones alternating with four non-bonding zones. Such an arrangement would permit random lateral aggregation of the macromolecules and also give electron dense bands at regular intervals. Thus, whilst there are still some points of contention, there is general agreement on the principles involved in collagen synthesis and these are summarized in *Fig: 28.*

So far we have discussed only the synthesis of collagen. However, on the basis of biochemical studies it is appreciated that connective tissue is capable of remodelling and turning over, and this obviously involves collagen. In simple terms it is best to imagine connective tissue in a steady state with the rate of collagen synthesis being balanced by the rate of collagen degradation: any change in the rates of either synthesis or degradation will result in either a net loss or gain of collagen. These rates vary from tissue to tissue and as we shall see (Chapter 19) the periodontal ligament probably has the highest rate of turnover of any connective tissue. As in the case of collagen synthesis, the manner in which collagen is degraded has not yet been fully elucidated. It has recently been established that the fibroblast plays a significant role in collagen degradation and

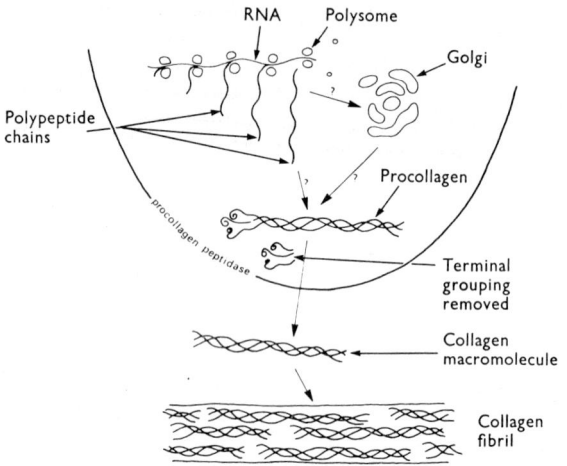

Fig. 28.—Collagen fibre formation. It is now known that in some cells the protein filaments pass through the Golgi apparatus before aggregating into procollagen.

that this cell is capable of phagocytosing collagen as well as synthesizing it. Thus it has been shown that the fibroblast can phagocytose collagen to form a phagosome (a vesicle containing the phagocytosed material) within the cell. This vesicle fuses with lysosomes and the collagen is degraded.

The above concept of connective tissue turnover and remodelling, namely simultaneous synthesis and degradation, is an important one. As has already been pointed out, any change in either rate of synthesis or degradation will lead to significant changes. For example, vitamin C deficiency interferes with intracellular collagen formation by preventing the hydroxylation of proline and lysine, but not with collagen breakdown. Thus, in the periodontal ligament, if collagen synthesis is halted by a deficiency of vitamin C, and degradation continues, a loss of collagen should be anticipated. This indeed occurs. So also with tooth movement. The remodelling of connective tissue required in this situation is most likely achieved

60

by the fibroblast but this has not, as yet, been demonstrated.

At the present time it is gradually being appreciated that not all collagen is exactly the same. Four genetically distinct collagens have so far been identified. Furthermore, each of these distinct types may differ in the types of cross-linkages developed thus bestowing different properties. Furthermore, when considering collagen in its biological context, as distinct from its chemistry, the immediate environment of the collagen fibril is also important. There is an intimate association between the collagen fibril and proteoglycans and variations in the latter significantly effect, it is thought, the behaviour of collagen in its tissue environment. Finally, it is now appreciated that some epithelial cells may synthesize collagen, including enamel epithelium.

REFERENCES

Deporter D. A. and Ten Cate A. R. (1973) Fine structural localization of acid and alkaline phosphatase in collagen-containing vesicles of fibroblasts. *J. Anat. Lond.* **114,** 457.

Eastoe J. E. (1968) Collagen and tissue architecture. *Dent. Pract. Dent. Rec.* **18,** 267.

Fitton J. S. (1968) The morphogenes of collagen. In: Gould B. S. (ed.), *Treatise on Collagen,* vol. 2, part B. New York, Academic, pp. 1–66.

Melcher A. H. and Eastoe J. E. (1969) The connective tissues of the periodontium. In: Melcher A. H. and Bowen W. H. (ed.), *The Biology of the Periodontium.* New York, Academic, pp. 176-343.

Olsen B. R. and Prokop D. J. (1974) Ferritin-conjugated antibodies used for labelling of organelles involved in the cellular synthesis and transport of procollagen. *Proc. Natl. Acad. Sci. U.S.A.* **71,** 2033.

Ross R. (1968) The connective tissue fibre-forming cell. In: Gould B. S. (ed.), *Treatise on Collagen,* vol. 2, part A. New York, Academic, pp. 2–82.

Trelstad R. L. and Slavkin H. C. (1974) Collagen synthesis by the epithelial enamel organ of the embryonic rabbit tooth. *Biochem. Biophys. Res. Commun.* **59,** 443.

Ten Cate A. R. (1972) Morphological studies of fibrocytes in connective tissue undergoing rapid remodelling. *J. Anat. Lond.* **112,** 401.

Ten Cate A. R. and Deporter D. A. (1975) The degradative role of the fibroblast in the remodelling and turnover of collagen in soft connective tissue. *Anat. Rec.* **182,** 1.

Weinstock M. and Leblond C. P. (1974) Formation of collagen. *Fed. Proc.* **33,** 1205.

CHAPTER 10

HARD TISSUE GENESIS

MOST accounts of hard tissue genesis deal specifically with a particular hard tissue and such accounts will also be found later in this book. The purpose of this chapter is to outline the factors common to the formation of all hard tissues and to emphasize the similarity of the principles involved in each, though the details of structure and composition may differ considerably.

When different forming hard tissues are studied it is readily apparent that there are many common features and these are represented in diagrammatic form in *Fig. 29*. Reference to this figure

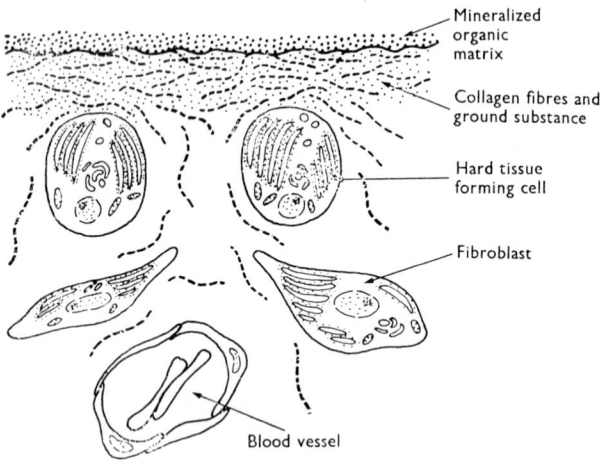

Fig. 29.—Diagram showing the essential features of hard tissue formation.

reveals that, in simple terms, hard tissue genesis involves the production of an organic matrix and the introduction into this matrix of mineral salts. The first step, therefore, in producing any hard tissue is to elaborate the organic matrix and for this a specialized cell is required. Such cells differentiate in areas of marked vascularity and have well defined characteristics. When compared with adjacent tissues these cells have more RNA, a higher oxidative enzyme activity and a higher hydrolytic enzyme activity. Ultrastructural features include a well developed 'rough' endoplasmic reticulum, Golgi apparatus, numerous mitochondria and secretory vesicles. These histochemical and ultrastructural features indicate that these cells are synthesizing and secreting material. Some of the aggregated proteins they secrete are built up extracellularly to form the fibrous component of the organic matrix. In addition these cells secrete the ground or cementing substance between the fibres which consists of mucopolysaccharides and glycoprotein.

Until quite recently the manner whereby mineral salts are introduced into an organic matrix was unknown. It was appreciated, however, that once the first crystals have been deposited in the organic matrix, further mineralization takes place by crystal growth. This led to the 'seeding' concept of mineralization. A good analogy is the well known experiment in which crystals are induced to grow by introducing dust particles into a super-saturated solution of copper sulphate: each dust particle acts as a nucleus of crystallization (epitactic focus). It has been shown *in vitro* that crystals can form spontaneously if the concentration of Ca and PO_4 ions is sufficiently high. However, sufficiently high concentrations are not found *in vivo* and hence there is a necessity for either some unknown nucleating substance to initiate crystal formation at the relatively low concentrations of Ca and PO_4 ions found in the body or for some mechanism to concentrate Ca and PO_4 ions locally. Recent structural and biochemical data indicate that the latter is the most likely mechanism. Electron microscopy has shown that at all sites, except those where mineralization is related to a pre-existing mineralized tissue (such as enamel on dentine and cement on dentine), cells bud off extracellular matrix vesicles and it is within these matrix vesicles that the needle-like apatite crystals are first seen. Perhaps these matrix vesicles provide the local mechanism for concentrating inorganic ions. How this is achieved is not known, but it is suggested that the matrix vesicles, which are rich with calcium-binding lipids, concentrate calcium and that alkaline phosphatase activity provides the local enrichment of phosphate ions.

A relationship between the activity of alkaline phosphatase and hard tissue formation has been recognized for over fifty years, yet its exact role is not at all certain. This is probably due to the fact that there are several alkaline phosphatases all working at differing pH ranges. Thus in addition to providing a local high phosphate ion concentration within matrix vesicles, it also seems very probable that activity of this enzyme is concerned with transporting calcium ions across cell membranes.

The marked activity of other hydrolytic enzymes (especially acid phosphatase) in cells forming hard tissues has not yet been related to any specific function. The fact that acid phosphatase activity is associated with catabolic events suggests that there is a rapid turnover of some cellular constituent(s).

Having outlined in fairly simple terms the salient features of hard tissue genesis, it is a rewarding exercise to examine the formation of the individual hard tissues to see how closely they are comparable. At the same time such a comparison should emphasize the similar principles involved in the genesis of each tissue.

Bones can be formed by either intramembranous or endochondral ossification. But the formation of actual bone tissue is fundamentally the same because, although in endochondral formation the bone is preceded by a cartilaginous model, this is replaced by bone deposited in the same way as in the intramembranous situation. Bone is mineralized connective tissue and its formation (intramembranous bone formation) is heralded by an increase in local vascularity of the mesenchyme. At the same time the cells of the mesenchyme in this area differentiate into distinctive cells called 'osteoblasts'. These cells are rich in RNA, associated with a well developed 'rough' endoplasmic reticulum, have a well developed Golgi apparatus and show high hydrolytic and oxidative enzyme activity. They synthesize the ground substance and the forerunners of the collagen macromolecule (procollagen) which is assembled extracellularly into collagen fibrils in the ground substance. The collagen fibrils and the ground substance constitute the organic matrix of unmineralized bone (osteoid), and it is into this that mineral salts are deposited. The first foci of mineral salts in the organic matrix are related to protoplasmic buds of the osteoblasts. Continued crystal growth from these foci results in the osteoblast becoming surrounded by mineralized matrix and the cell is then termed an 'osteocyte'.

Fig. 30 illustrates this sequence of events and it will be seen that it is essentially similar to *Fig. 29*, differing only in that the bone-forming cells become trapped within the forming hard tissue. In endochondral bone formation the cartilage model is invaded by vascular mesenchymal osteogenic tissue which elaborates bone in essentially the same manner as outlined above. However, there is one significant difference: when the cartilage model is invaded by osteogenic tissue the cartilage mineralizes, and this mineralized cartilage provides the scaffold for the forming bone. In this situation the newly formed osteoid does not seem to mineralize by the provision of epitactic foci in the form of matrix vesicles. Instead, mineralization occurs by crystal growth from the pre-existing crystallites in the mineralized cartilage. It must be pointed out that this account of bone formation applies to the formation of embryonic bone. The coarse-fibred embryonic bone later undergoes remodelling to be replaced by adult fine-fibred bone.

The mode of formation of cement is almost identical to that of bone. Cement is also a mineralized connective tissue and is formed by cementoblasts, the cement-forming cells, which differentiate from the ectomesenchymal dental follicle surrounding the developing root. These cells exhibit high hydrolytic enzyme activity, oxidative enzyme activity, and have a well developed 'rough' endoplasmic reticulum and Golgi apparatus. They elaborate the collagen fibrils of the unmineralized cement matrix (cementoid). The cementoblasts may

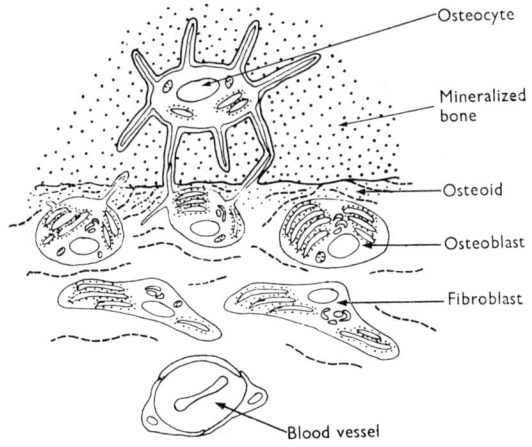

Fig. 30.—Osteogenesis.

or may not be incorporated in the mineralizing matrix and this determines the two types of cement seen in histological sections, acellular and cellular. *Fig. 31* gives the essential details of cemento-genesis. As cement is laid down over the pre-existing dentine, the

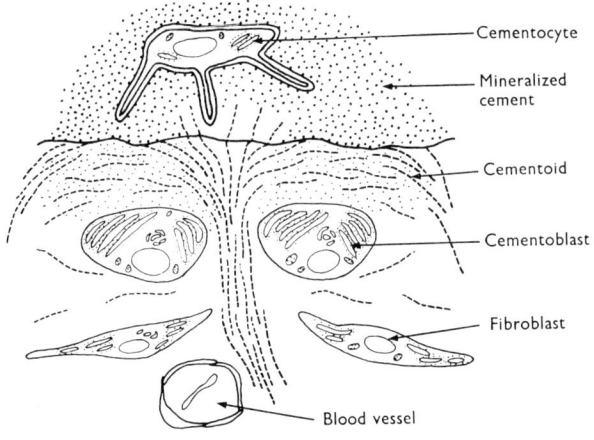

Fig. 31.—Cementogenesis.

initial mineralization of the cementoid takes place by crystal growth from the mineralized dentine.

Like cement, dentine is also formed from ectomesenchymal connective tissue but it differs significantly from bone and cement, especially in its structural features. Even so, the principles underlying its formation are the same. Specialized cells, the odontoblasts, differentiate from the cells of the dental papilla due to induction by the cells of the internal enamel epithelium. At the same time other papillary cells congregate beneath the newly differentiated odontoblasts, forming the sub-odontoblast layer (*Fig. 32*) between which are the vessels of the sub-odontoblast capillary plexus. The newly differentiated odontoblasts develop an extensive endoplasmic reticulum, a prominent Golgi apparatus, and exhibit marked oxidative and hydrolytic enzyme activity apart from alkaline phosphatase. This enzyme is found initially in the cells of the sub-odontoblast layer and it is from this layer that large fibre bundles, the fibres of von Korff, originate.

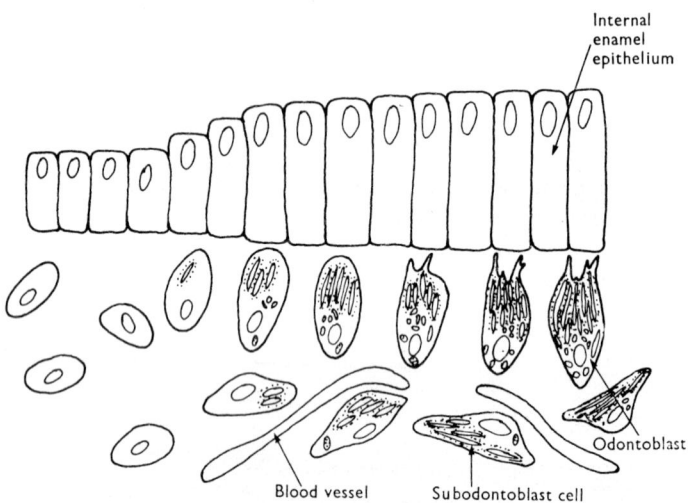

Fig. 32.—Differentiation of odontoblasts.

These fibres pass between the odontoblasts and fan out close to the basement membrane of the internal enamel epithelium and together with the ground substance form the organic matrix of dentine (*Fig. 33*). While the organic matrix is being formed, the odontoblasts retreat towards the centre of the papilla, each leaving behind a slender process which becomes surrounded by matrix. The dentine matrix becomes mineralized to form tubular dentine (*Fig. 34*). The odontoblasts in this situation, like the osteoblasts in membranous ossification, have cellular buds which become matrix vesicles and most likely provide the foci for mineralization.

This sequence of events only applies to the very first dentine (mantle dentine) elaborated against the internal enamel epithelium.

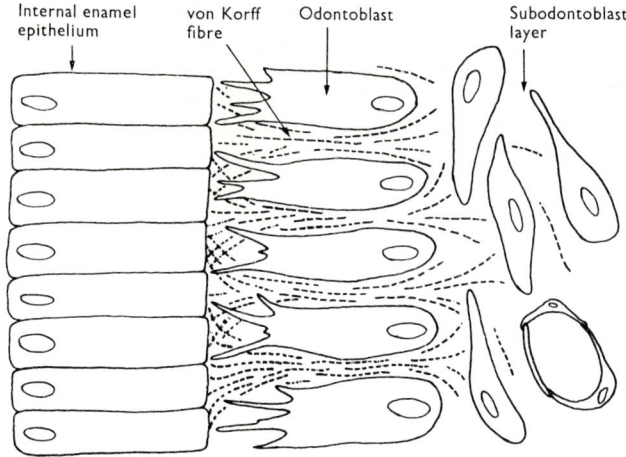

Fig. 33.—The origin and distribution of classic von Korff fibres.

After this first increment of dentine forms, the fibrous component for the remainder of the matrix is manufactured by the odontoblasts (*Fig. 35*). It is significant that when this switch in the origin of the fibrous matrix occurs there is a reduction in the number of von

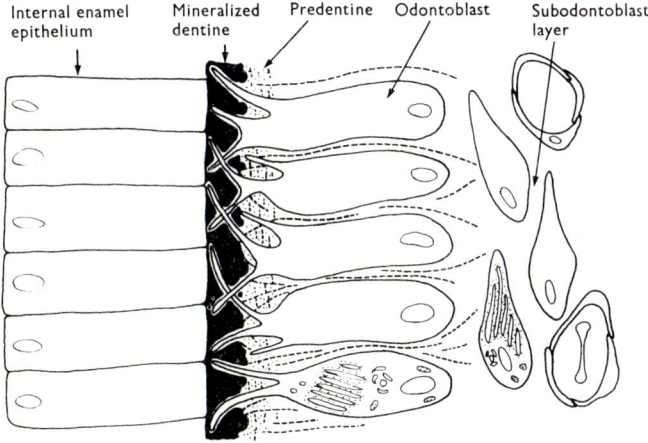

Fig. 34.—Starting the formation of dentinal tubules.

67

Korff fibres and that the enzyme alkaline phosphatase now becomes demonstrable within the odontoblasts. This widely accepted account of dentinogenesis is correct in principle. However, recent studies have queried whether von Korff fibres really exist and these studies will be discussed fully in the chapter on dentinogenesis.

Thus far, therefore, it is evident that osteogenesis, cementogenesis, and dentinogenesis have many common features. These hard tissues are all specialized forms of connective tissue, they all develop in areas of high vascularity; specialized cells are associated with the formation of the organic matrix which consists of collagen fibrils

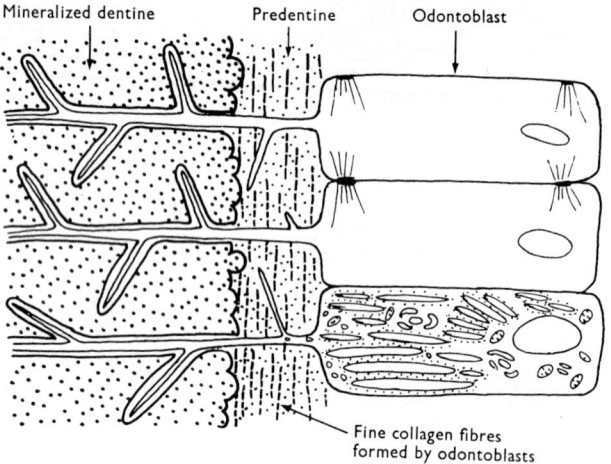

Fig. 35.—Circumpulpal dentinogenesis.

and a ground substance. The cells have common ultrastructural and enzymatic features and mineralization occurs within the organic matrix.

When amelogenesis is considered it would appear that enamel formation differs significantly from that of the other hard tissues. Enamel is an epidermal product and for this reason its organic matrix does not contain collagen. By analogy with the fibrous collagen scaffolding of other mesenchymal hard tissues it was once assumed that enamel employed a fibrous keratin to fulfil the same function. However, this is now thought not to be the case and, although no fibrous component is involved in enamel matrix formation, amelogenesis can be shown to be closely similar in principle to the formation of other hard tissues.

The histology of amelogenesis, outlined in *Fig. 36*, shows that two cellular elements are involved, the enamel forming cells or amelo-blasts, and the cells of the stratum intermedium. The latter are exceptionally rich in alkaline phosphatase activity and the amelo-blasts are rich in RNA and have a high activity of oxidative enzymes. If the ultrastructure of the ameloblast is examined, its features are essentially similar to those of the osteoblast or odontoblast in that there is a well developed 'rough' endoplasmic reticulum, Golgi apparatus, many mitochondria and secretory vesicles. In other words, it has the characteristics of a protein synthesizing and secreting cell.

In view of the once supposed presence of keratinous material in enamel matrix, it is interesting to compare the ultrastructure of the ameloblast with that of the keratin producing cell. The keratinizing cell has very little 'rough' endoplasmic reticulum but instead has many free ribosomes. The protein synthesized in this cell is retained and aggregated in a fibrous form, so that the cytoplasm eventually becomes laden with keratin. Such a cell is described as a protein-

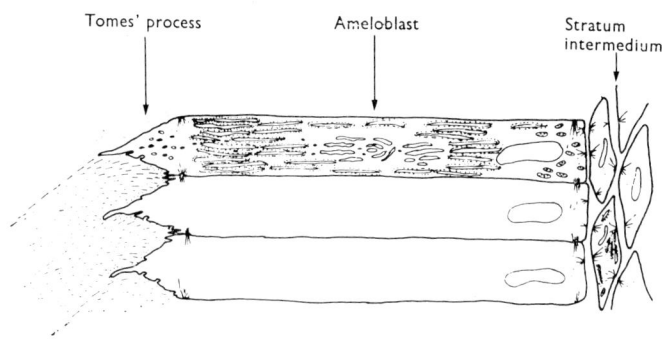

Fig. 36.—Amelogenesis.

synthesizing and retaining cell and it is clear from a comparison between *Fig. 8* (p. 16) and *Fig. 36* that the ameloblast does not fall into this category. Thus far amelogenesis corresponds to the genesis of the other hard tissues. Blood vessels are present, adjacent to the outer enamel epithelium, the enzymatic picture corresponds and the formative cell secretes a proteinaceous material which forms the organic matrix. However, when discussing amelogenesis later in this book, evidence will be presented showing that this organic matrix does not become organized into a fibrous form but remains in the form of a gel. Into this organic matrix mineral salts are deposited. There is no evidence for any matrix vesicles associated with the ameloblast and it is thought that initial mineralization of enamel starts by crystal growth from the mineralized dentine which supports the first formed enamel matrix.

It is apparent, then, that the hard tissues, irrespective of their derivation, reveal similar principles in their genesis. These may be summarized as the production of an organic matrix by cells which exhibit protein synthesizing and secreting features, and introduction into this matrix of mineral salts.

It is useful to summarize here this new concept of mineralization of hard tissues. The suggestion is that where mineralization is occurring for the first time, such as in membranous bone formation, dentine formation and in mineralizing cartilage, the foci for the initial appearance of inorganic crystals are buds or extensions of the cell associated with deposition of the organic matrix. Where hard tissue genesis is taking place in association with pre-existing mineralized tissue, for example cement in relation to mineralized dentine, bone in relation to mineralized cartilage and enamel in relation to mineralized dentine, mineralization occurs in the newly formed matrix by crystal growth from the pre-existing mineralized tissue.

REFERENCES

References pertinent to this chapter can be found following the Chapters on Dentinogenesis, Amelogenesis, and Cementogenesis.

CHAPTER 11

BONE

THIS chapter does not attempt to deal with the detailed histology of bone for which the reader is referred to any standard histology textbook. Rather we present one or two aspects of bone not normally considered in such sources but which are of some significance in clarifying terminology and explaining such phenomena as tooth movement and facial growth.

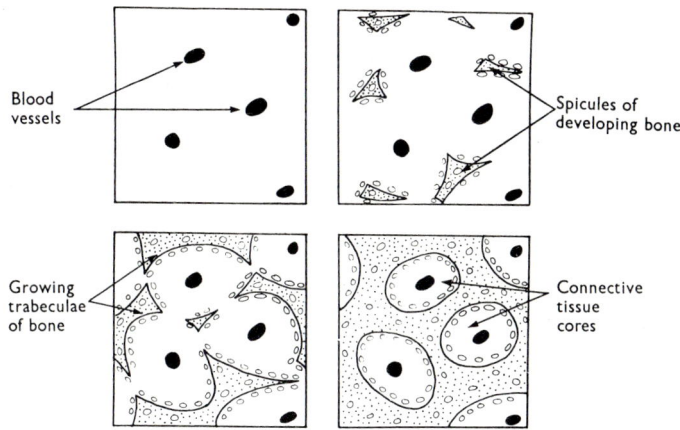

Fig. 37.—Four stages in the formation of embryonic (woven, immature, coarse-fibred) bone.

When bone tissue is first formed, or when it is rapidly laid down, for example in the embryo and in the repair of wounds, the pre-existing connective tissue of the area is colonized by new bone. The collagen in the connective tissue and the collagen elaborated by the newly differentiated bone forming cells, the osteoblasts, together form the fibrous matrix of this new bone. As a result the collagen fibres are of varying thickness and orientation and many are continuous with the collagen fibres of the adjacent soft connective tissue. This type of bone is termed 'coarse fibred woven bone' or 'embryonic bone' and is laid down in trabeculae or plates which surround areas of soft connective tissue (*Fig. 37*).

From this starting point woven bone is remodelled to form mature bone. In mature bone the collagen fibres of the matrix are of even

71

thickness and are laid down in sheets or lamellae. In each lamella the collagen fibres are all orientated in one direction, although the orientation and number of collagen fibres varies from lamella to lamella. Lamellae of bone are laid down in two ways. They can be laid down concentrically (from outside to inside) to form osteons (Haversian systems) or in sheets on the surface of bones as circumferential lamellae. Embryonic bone is replaced by mature bone as follows. Between the trabeculae of woven bone is soft connective tissue with its associated blood vessels. On the internal surface of the trabeculae new bone is laid down in layers of lamellae with the result that, as each layer is laid down, the volume of the unmineralized connective tissue is diminished until only a small core, which transmits blood vessels, remains. This osteon formed within woven bone is termed a 'primary' osteon (*Fig. 38*). The primary osteon

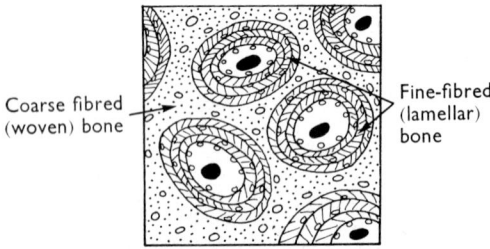

Coarse fibred (woven) bone

Fine-fibred (lamellar) bone

Fig. 38.—Primary osteons form within the trabeculae of woven bone.

has a periphery which is ill-defined when viewed in the light microscope because the collagen fibres here are continuous with those of the woven bone. Also the cells in woven bone are larger and have an irregular disposition. Thus we now have a form of bone which consists of a mixture of woven bone, primary osteons, and circumferential bone at its periphery.

From this point on, either mature compact (adult) bone or mature cancellous (adult) bone is developed. These two types of bone can be distinguished by their ratios of hard and soft connective tissue. Thus compact bone consists of comparatively solid blocks of bone in which the proportion of mineralized tissue is far greater than the proportion of soft connective tissue, whereas in cancellous bone the blocks of bone are separated by a considerable portion of soft connective tissue and macroscopically have a honeycomb appearance. Mature bone is formed by a process of careful remodelling whereas resorption first takes place indiscriminately within the trabeculae of primary osteons and woven bone. The area resorbed is replaced by soft connective tissue. Within the concavity of the resorbed area bone is laid down, in a similar manner as described for the primary osteon, to form what is termed the 'secondary osteon' (*Fig. 39*). The secondary osteon is marked at its periphery by a reversal line which indicates the extent of resorption. Depending on the amount of remodelling and infilling of the soft connective tissue spaces, either mature cancellous or mature compact bone is formed. During remodelling, remnants of previous osteons remain and these are termed 'interstitial bone'.

It must be realized that the above account is somewhat simplified and transitional forms of bone are often seen. In summary, however, we can consider compact bone as consisting of surface or circumferential lamellar bone, primary and secondary (tertiary and so on) osteons and interstitial bone—the latter consisting of either remnants of previous osteons or of parts of other osteons. The relative amounts of each vary considerably in samples of compact bone from different

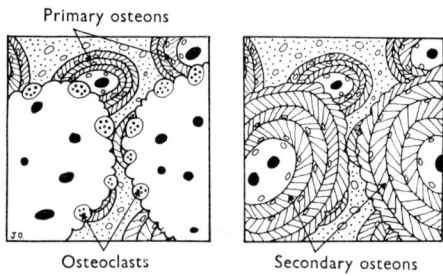

Primary osteons

Osteoclasts   Secondary osteons

Fig. 39.—The conversion of embryonic bone into adult bone; the formation of secondary osteons.

sources. Cancellous or trabecular bone has a similar structure to compact bone but differs in that complete osteons are fewer and there is a much greater amount of interstitial bone.

This account of bone development should make an understanding of bone terminology a little easier. This terminology is somewhat confusing because of the several different ways of classifying bone. *Fig. 40* summarizes the ways in which bone has been classified. The table explains why fine fibred lamellar bone is found in Haversian system bone and in compact bone; why Haversian system bone is found in cancellous bone. A simple way to remember the differing classifications of bone is to relate each classification to an order of magnification, namely with the naked eye, with a low power lens and with a high power lens.

From the above account it is evident, therefore, that a considerable amount of internal remodelling by means of resorption and deposition occurs within bone.

The remodelling of surface bone plays a significant part in bone growth. Surface remodelling is brought about in the same way as internal remodelling, namely by means of controlled sites of bone deposition and bone resorption utilizing the same cellular bases, the osteoblast and the osteoclast.

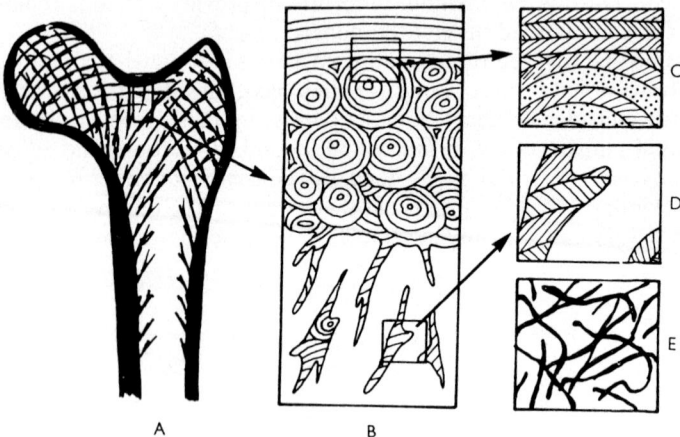

Fig. 40.—Some terms used in the description of bone tissue. A, Viewed with the naked eye bone appears to be either compact or cancellous (= spongy or trabecular). The compact layer forms the cortex of the bone; hence the term 'cortical bone'. B, Viewed with a low power lens the deeper region of the compact (= cortical) bone is seen to consist of Haversian systems (= osteons) in which layers (= lamellae) of bone are arranged concentrically around each central canal of the system. At the periphery of the compact layer, the lamellae are arranged circumferentially around the surface of the whole bone. Therefore compact bone contains concentric, circumferential and, in the spaces, interstitial lamellae. It will be noted that the trabeculae in spongy bone are also composed of lamellae. All (nearly) the bone in an adult is built up of lamellae (C, D) in which the collagen fibres are regular and fine. In adjacent lamellae the fibres run in different directions (some fibres are often cut transversely, appearing as dots in a section: C). Therefore, adult bone is both fine-fibred and lamellated. In contrast, woven (= embryonic) bone contains coarse, irregularly arranged fibres (E).

An appreciation of both the nature and extent of bone remodelling explains its remarkable plasticity seen during development. The constant deposition and removal of bone tissue, again and again, accommodates the growth of a bone without changing its shape, function or relation to neighbouring structures. Thus, for example, a significant increase in size of the mandible is achieved from birth to maturity largely by bony remodelling without any loss in function or change in its relative position in the maxilla. It is most unlikely that any of the bone tissue present in the 1 year old mandible is present in the same bone thirty years later.

REFERENCES

For further reading on the structure and function of bone the three volumes of *The Biochemistry and Physiology of Bone*, edited by G. H. Bourne (New York, Academic, 1972) and *The Physiology of Bone* by J. M. Vaughan (Oxford, Clarendon Press, 1970) are recommended.

CHAPTER 12

DENTINOGENESIS

THE formation of dentine begins at the late bell stage of tooth development and is a function of the dental papilla. Immediately before the start of dentinogenesis changes are found within the cells of the internal enamel epithelium. The short columnar cells of this epithelium become tall columnar and their nuclei move to the ends of the cells away from the papilla. Tissue culture studies have shown unequivocally that these elongated cells organize the differentiation of the peripheral cells of the dental papilla into odontoblasts. However, in terms of induction, the significance of these morphological changes in the internal enamel epithelium may have been overemphasized because a similar induction of papilla cells takes place during root formation without the equivalent epithelial cells undergoing these changes.

The newly differentiated odontoblast is characterized histologically by its location and its size; histochemically by its high RNA content and marked oxidative and hydrolytic enzyme activity. This latter characteristic must be qualified in that although increase in acid phosphatase and non-specific esterase can be demonstrated, the newly differentiated odontoblast does not possess alkaline phosphatase activity at a level which can be visualized by light microscopy. Ultrastructurally this cell exhibits a well developed 'rough' endoplasmic reticulum; Golgi apparatus; numerous mitochondria, some of which contain alkaline phosphatase activity; many vesicular structures; and a well developed micro-tubular system. At the same time as the odontoblasts differentiate there is an increase in the number of the immediately subjacent cells of the papilla which become a recognizable subodontoblast layer. A feature of the cells of this layer is a high alkaline phosphatase activity associated with their cell membranes. Ground substance fills the extracellular compartment which also contains a capillary plexus (*Fig. 41*).

The next step in the generally accepted account of formation of dentine is the production of collagen by the cellular elements of the sub-odontoblast layer. The collagen molecules link together extracellularly so that distinct fibre bundles can be recognized at this time in silver stained sections examined with the light microscope (*Fig. 42*). These fibre bundles, the fibres of von Korff, appear to spiral between the odontoblasts and are described as 'fanning out' against the surface of the basement lamina of the internal enamel

76

epithelium where they form the fibrillar component of the organic matrix of the first formed dentine. Simultaneously with the formation of the von Korff fibres, the odontoblasts and sub-odontoblast cells move away from the basement membrane. As they do so,

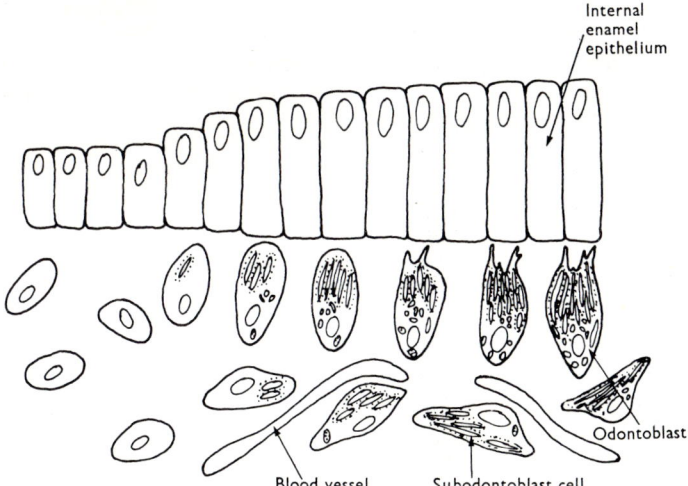

Fig. 41.—Diagram illustrating the progressive differentiation of odontoblasts from left to right.

the odontoblasts each leave behind one or more slender cytoplasmic odontoblast processes which eventually lie within a dentine tubule when the dentine matrix becomes mineralized (*Fig. 43*).

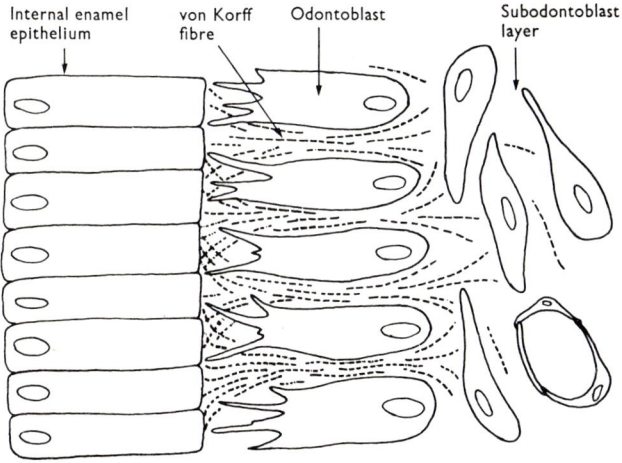

Fig. 42.—The formation of classic von Korff fibres.

The ground substance of the dentine matrix may either be contributed by acid mucopolysaccharides from the dental papilla which becomes progressively smaller with continued dentine formation or alternatively, and more likely, be secreted by odontoblasts. Thus, the von Korff fibres and the ground substance together form the organic matrix of the dentine which, in its non-mineralized state is termed 'predentine'. It must be appreciated that during dentinogenesis there is always a layer of predentine into which mineral salts are deposited.

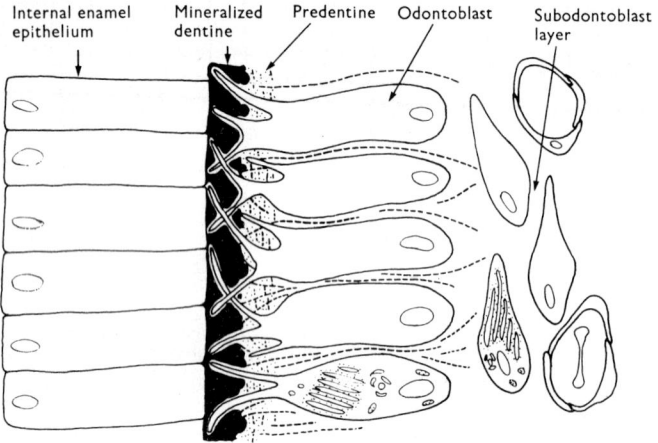

Fig. 43.—Starting the formation of dentinal tubules.

The foregoing applies to the first dentine formed in the tooth germ and later dentinogenesis differs in some aspects of its formation. It has long been known that the dentine immediately below the enamel, the first formed dentine, differs from the bulk of the dentine in having an organic matrix with coarse collagen fibres. Thus, mantle dentine (the first formed) and circumpulpal dentine (the bulk of the dentine) are recognized. Evidence for the difference of their fibre content is based, in part, on the fact that there are fewer von Korff 'fibres' in sections of circumpulpal dentinogenesis and that electron microscopy and autoradiographic studies have established that the odontoblast elaborates the fine fibred collagen of the circumpulpal dentine.

On the basis of recent work, however, this account of dentine formation is incorrect in some details. Thus the contribution of the so-called 'von Korff fibres' must be questioned. It has been shown that von Korff fibres are structures seen only with the light microscope. When thick sections of a developing tooth (50 μm) are stained with silver and examined with the light microscope the classic picture of many argyrophilic (silver-loving) von Korff fibres related to initial dentinogenesis and few to later dentinogenesis is seen. If this same thick section is now thin sectioned and examined with the electron microscope, von Korff fibres cannot be identified (*Fig. 44*). Instead, the stain is seen as small particles of silver in an extensive extracellular compartment, between the newly differentiated odontoblasts, which contains no banded collagen. Furthermore, if sections are pretreated with acetic anhydride which blocks reducing sugars, no silver staining of the sections occurs. This suggests that the silver had been captured by the reducing sugars of the ground substances. How then can these observations be correlated with the presence of von Korff fibres? Presumably the extensive intercellular compartment between the newly differentiated odontoblasts contains reducing sugars which can become impregnated with silver. When viewed with the light microscope, the resultant negative outline of the odontoblasts simulates the appearance of fibres (*Fig. 45*). This explanation of the so-called 'von Korff fibres' also accounts for their diminution as circumpulpal dentinogenesis begins. As the odontoblasts hypertrophy, they became more closely packed together, develop tight junctions and eliminate most of the extracellular compartment between them (*Fig. 46.*). Hence there can be no extracellular deposition of silver and no 'von Korff fibres'. Thus, a dual origin for the fibre component of dentine matrix must be disputed.

It is still necessary, however, to explain why there is a difference in the fibrous matrix of mantle and circumpulpal dentine with mantle dentine containing coarse collagen fibres and circumpulpal dentine fine collagen fibres. On the basis of autoradiographic studies it is now almost certain that the odontoblasts synthesize and secrete all dentine collagen. Clearly, the very first formed collagen is aggregated in a different environment from later-formed collagen. The first formed collagen is aggregated within an extracellular compartment with abundant ground substance, whereas in later dentinogenesis the collagen is aggregated in an environment of minimal ground substance (*Fig. 47*). It is possible that the larger extracellular compartment which exist's at the beginning of dentinogenesis permits aggregation of large fibre bundles. It is certainly the case that large fibre bundles can be seen related to early dentine formation, but always at the neck of the odontoblast and not between these cells.

For 40 years the activity of the enzyme alkaline phosphatase has been noted in relation to dentinogenesis and, for that matter, to the genesis of other hard tissues also. It has been suggested that its activity is related to either mineralization, ground substance synthesis or collagen synthesis. Recent fine structural studies of the localization of alkaline phosphatase activity during dentinogenesis are of interest and clarify this problem slightly. Enzyme activity first occurs in association with the cell membrane of the cells of the presumptive sub-odontoblast layer. As the odontoblast differentiates, enzyme activity becomes demonstrable at the odontoblast cell

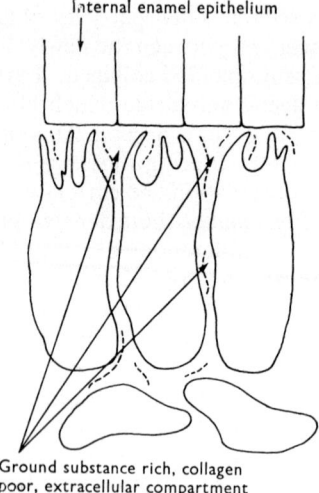

Internal enamel epithelium

Ground substance rich, collagen poor, extracellular compartment

Fig. 44.—Electron microscope appearance of the extracellular space between newly differentiated odontoblasts.

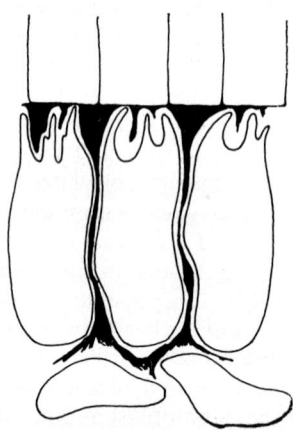

Fig. 45.—Silver stains 'lake' in the extracellular compartment giving it the appearance of fibres when viewed with the light microscope. C.f. *Fig. 44.*

surface and also in association with the matrix vesicles in the predentine matrix. The localization of enzyme activity at the cell membrane may be equated with calcium transport and its location in matrix vesicles with the production of a high concentration of phosphate ions (*see* Chapter 10). Fine structural localization of enzyme activity has provided no real evidence that it is related to either ground substance or collagen synthesis.

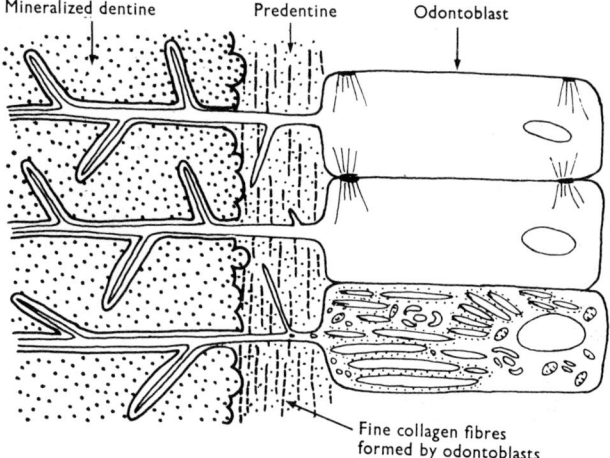

Fig. 46.—Circumpulpal dentinogenesis.

Examination of the fine structure of dentine reveals the presence of a sheath of more highly mineralized peritubular dentine around the odontoblast process (*Fig. 48*). The first appearance of the peritubular dentine is in the fully mineralized dentine matrix near the

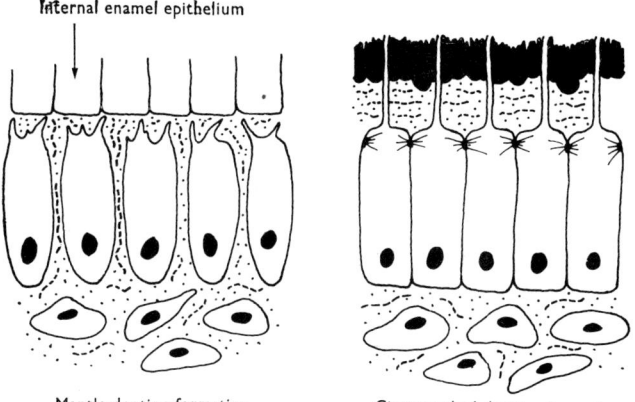

Fig. 47.—The essential differences between the formation of mantle dentine and circumpulpal dentine. In the latter the tightly packed odontoblasts prevent pulpal material being incorporated into the predentine.

81

predentine–dentine border, and coincides with the narrowing in width of the odontoblast process; the peritubular dentine thus occupies some of the space formerly occupied by the odontoblast process. Little is known about the genesis of the peritubular dentine. However, there are certain features of the odontoblast, its process and the peri-tubular dentine which permit some speculation.

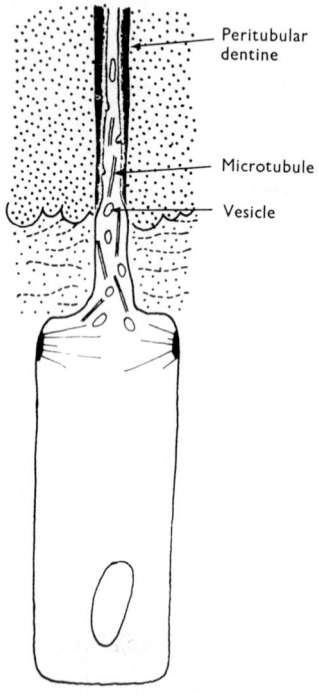

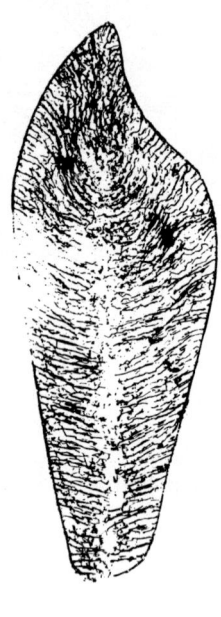

Fig. 48.—Diagram showing the formation of peri-tubular dentine.

Fig. 49.—Scratch marks made on smoked card by beads simulating the primary curvatures of dentine tubules.

There are morphological features of the odontoblast and its process which can be equated, in part, with synthesis of the peritubular dentine. Thus, the odontoblast process contains a well developed system of micro-tubules, vesicular structures and surface bays, which have, in other situations, been equated with transport and secretory mechanisms. The presence of such structures within the odontoblast process explains how peritubular dentine might be formed within the depths of already formed dentine. Material synthesized by the odontoblast cell body could pass via the process to the site of peritubular dentine formation.

However, the above features might merely demonstrate activity of odontoblasts unrelated to the development of peritubular dentine. In this case, peritubular dentine formation would involve a redistribution of dentine mineral in response to purely physico-chemical changes.

Another interesting aspect of dentinogenesis is the course taken by the odontoblasts as they retreat towards the centre of the pulp. As they leave behind them a process which is incorporated in the mineralized matrix, examination of the tubules of mature dentine provides a permanent record of the path taken by the individual odontoblasts. It is known that the odontoblast processes have a primary 'S' shaped curvature and also secondary curvatures.

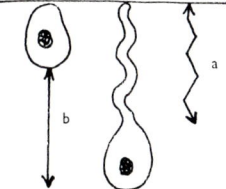

Fig. 50.—Distance, a, the true length of the forming odontoblast process, is greater than b, the distance moved by the odontoblast in the same time.

There is a hypothesis to explain the genesis of these curvatures It has been suggested that the primary curvatures result from the oscillations of the odontoblasts which arise from their crowding as the volume of the pulp decreases. This has been tested by a simple model experiment. The outline of the dentine surface of a tooth in longitudinal section is traced on smoked paper. If beads, representing the odontoblasts, are aligned along the periphery of the drawing and progressively pushed in a centripetal direction, starting with those beneath the cusp tip, the sinuous tracks so produced on the smoked paper mimic the primary curvatures of the dentinal tubules (*Fig. 49*). At the same time, it will be seen that the beads become progressively more crowded as they move centri-petally. The origin of the secondary curvatures is more difficult to explain, but a tentative solution has been offered. This is based upon the accepted observation that enamel spindles are most fre-quently encountered beneath the tips of cusps, where crowding of the retreating odontoblasts is most intense. Under such conditions, it is suggested that in unit time the formed length of the odontoblast process is greater than the distance moved by the odontoblast towards the papilla (*Fig. 50*). Hence, the process might become buckled and the secondary curvatures established.

REFERENCES

Eisenmann D. R. and Glick P. L. (1972) Ultrastructure of initial crystal formation in dentine. *J. Ult. Res.* **41**, 18.

Garant P. R., Zabo G. and Nalbandian J. (1968) The fine structure of the mouse odontoblast. *Archs Oral Biol.* **13**, 857.

Harrop T. J. and Mackay B. (1968) Electron microscopic observations on healing in the dental pulp in the rat. *Archs Oral Biol.* **13**, 365.

Herold R. C. and Kaye H. (1966) Mitochondria in odontoblastic processes. *Nature, Lond.* **210**, 108.

Lester K. S. and Boyde A. (1968) The question of von Korff fibres in mammalian dentine. *Calc. Tiss. Res.* **1**, 273.

Melcher A. H. and Eastoe J. E. (1969) The connective tissues of the periodontium. In: Melcher A. H. and Bowen W. H. (ed.), *The Biology of the Periodontium.* New York, Academic, pp. 176–343.

Noble H. W., Carmichael A. F. and Rankine H. (1962) Electron microscopy of human developing dentine. *Archs Oral Biol.* **7**, 395.

Osborn J. W. (1967) A mechanistic view of dentinogenesis and its relation to the curvatures of the processes of the odontoblasts. *Archs Oral Biol.* **12**, 275.

Reith E. J. (1968) Collagen formation in developing molar teeth of rats. *J. Ult. Res.* **21**, 383.

Sisca R. F. and Provenza D. V. (1972) Initial dentine formation in human deciduous teeth. An electron microscope study. *Calc. Tiss. Res.* **9**, 1.

Symons N. B. B. (1956) The development of the fibres of the dentine matrix. *Br. dent. J.* **101**, 252.

Symons N. B. B. (1962) A histochemical study of the odontoblast process. *Archs Oral Biol.* **7**, 455.

Ten Cate A. R. (1962) The distribution of alkaline phosphatase in the human tooth germ. *Archs Oral Biol.* **7**, 195.

Ten Cate A. R. (1966) Alkaline phosphatase activity and the formation of human circumpulpal dentine. *Archs Oral Biol.* **11**, 267.

Ten Cate A. R. (1968) Current concepts and problems of dentinogenesis. In: Symons N. B. B. (ed.), *Dentine and Pulp.* Edinburgh, Livingstone, pp. 9–18.

Ten Cate A. R., Melcher A. H., Pudy G. and Wagner D. (1970) The non-fibrous nature of the von Korff fibres in developing dentine. A light and electron microscopic study. *Anat. Rec.* **168**, 491.

Yoshiki S. and Kurahashi Y. (1971) A light and electron microscopic study of alkaline phosphatase activity in the early stages of dentinogenesis in the young rat. *Archs Oral Biol.* **16**, 1143.

CHAPTER 13

THE STRUCTURE OF DENTINE

WELL documented accounts of dentine structure are available in the standard dental texts and no useful purpose would be served by repeating their contents. There are, however, certain structural features which have recently been investigated and it is the purpose of this chapter to present these to the reader. Some of these features are represented diagrammatically in *Fig. 51*.

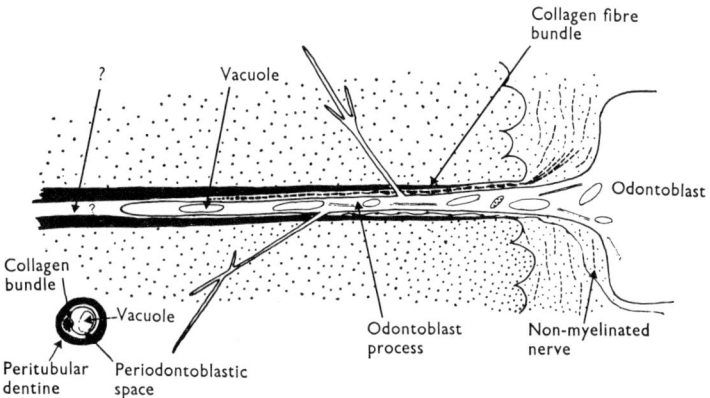

Fig. 51.—Some of the structures related to odontoblast processes.

The layer of dentine adjacent to the enamel (mantle dentine) differs from the bulk of the dentine (circumpulpal dentine) in the configuration of the collagen fibres of the matrix. Classically the thick fibres of von Korff are thought to provide the fibre content of the mantle dentine matrix and, apart from where they fan out at the enamel dentine junction, to be parallel to the dentinal tubules. The matrix fibres of circumpulpal dentine are much finer and weave across each other at right angles to the tubules. As von Korff fibres can be seen between odontoblasts forming circumpulpal dentine it might seem that these fibres should be visible in mineralized circumpulpal dentine. However, such fibres are only rarely seen and it has been suggested that these thick fibres become split and re-orientated at right angles to the tubules during circumpulpal dentinogenesis. However, in view of the recent findings concerning von Korff fibres discussed in the previous chapter their contribution must be reassessed. It is clear from *Fig. 47* (*see* p. 81) that while mantle dentine is being formed a good deal of ground substance-rich, collagen-poor extracellular material is incorporated, whereas little ground substance is incorporated into the circumpulpal dentine matrix. There is, therefore, a real difference in the formation of the matrices of mantle and circumpulpal dentine.

The capricious demonstration of von Korff fibres during circumpulpal dentinogenesis at the light microscope level can be explained on the basis of the separation of some odontoblasts, the majority of which, when seen with the electron microscope, are closely packed and united by means of tight junctions. Silver which has been deposited between the separate odontoblasts will be seen as von Korff fibres with the light microscope. In the subsurface zone of the root dentine the finer fibres are curved and said to be arranged in 'arcades'. It is possible that as the calcospherites form they mould the fibres into these arcades which are then stabilized by the ensuing mineralization.

The highly mineralized peritubular dentine is generally thickest on the side of the tubule towards the occlusal surface of the tooth. Most studies have suggested that the matrix of peritubular dentine consists of very sparse fine collagen fibres, although it has also been suggested that this region is devoid of any fibrous material, thus giving it affinities with enamel. Recent electron microscope studies show that there is a space between the odontoblast process and the tubule wall; this space is termed the 'periodontoblastic' space (*Fig. 51*). These same studies showed that the space was occupied by an amorphous ground substance containing occasional fine non-mineralized collagen fibres, which may or may not become incorporated in the hypermineralized peritubular dentine. Electron micrographs have recently shown the presence of one or more thick non-mineralized collagen fibres running beside the odontoblast process within the dentinal tubule (*Fig. 51*). Though their presence is as yet unexplained, it might be that they are produced by aggregation of the fine collagen fibres just mentioned.

From time to time cytoplasmic vacuoles within the odontoblasts have been described. Recent electron microscopic studies show that these vacuoles are also present within the odontoblast process, being relatively small and quite numerous at the pulpal end (*Fig. 51*). The contents of the vacuoles appear finely stippled under the electron microscope and this material is thought to be discharged into the periodontoblastic space by a process of reverse pinocytosis. However, the chemical nature of the vacuole contents has not yet been investigated. At these high magnifications, the cytoplasm of the most terminal end of the odontoblast processes has a hyaline appearance (*see next paragraph*). Recent histochemical studies show the presence of hydrolytic enzymes and lipid, represented in particulate form, within the odontoblast process and the lateral processes. Their localization may possibly correspond with the vacuolar structures seen in electron micrographs suggesting that the odontoblast process is not merely an inactive cell extension. A few mitochondria have now been demonstrated in the odontoblast process within the mineralized dentine (*Fig. 51*). This finding has been confirmed by the demonstration of oxidative enzymes within the odontoblast process. Numerous microtubules and fine filaments are also present in the odontoblast processes, but their function is unknown, although it has been suggested that they provide pathways for metabolites.

All the above are based upon descriptions from several studies on differing mammalian species. A recent investigation with the scanning electron microscope of human dentine has produced some unusual and startling findings and is therefore worth quoting extensively. Young permanent premolars were fractured and the fracture surfaces prepared for study by scanning electron microscopy. With this method it was found that the odontoblast process occupies a tubule only a quarter of its total extent from the pulp and that all tubules at a distance from the pulp of more than 0·7 mm are quite empty (*Fig. 51*).

These observations have been confirmed by a study of dentine from the cat which has clearly shown that the peripheral half of the dentinal tubules contains no cellular material. The earlier failure to 'recognize' the absence of cytoplasmic processes in the outer half of fully formed dentine is probably due to the difficulty in cutting sections of this tissue for electronmicroscopy: previous studies have generally been confined to regions very close to the predentine, a region which is easier to section.

The apparent lack of odontoblast cell process in tubules up to the dentino-enamel junction has obvious implications in any discussion of dentine sensitivity. If an odontoblast cell process is absent from three quarters of its tubule the question arises as to what occupies the tubule. It has been suggested that the tubule is filled with extra-cellular fluid.

Microscopic examination of ground sections of dentine reveals the presence of interglobular dentine, most frequently beneath the enamel–dentine junction. These three-dimensional spaces are interpreted as areas of deficient mineralization of the dentine matrix, representing the interstices between calcospherites which have failed to fuse completely. It has been shown, however, that the interstitial spaces visualized in stained decalcified sections are more numerous than the areas of interglobular dentine seen in microradiographs of ground sections. In general the dentinal tubules extend uninterruptedly through the interglobular spaces, although it has been suggested that sometimes the tubules themselves expand to become the spaces. Peritubular dentine is not found in interglobular spaces. From this it might be argued that mineralized intertubular dentine must be present before peritubular dentine can be developed. However, in some animals peritubular dentine forms in the region of the predentine; that is, before the intertubular dentine is mineralized. This suggests that the mineralization of dentine may be under the control of the odontoblast processes rather than being a simple physico-chemical reaction of mature dentine matrix. In the absence of the control, not only does intertubular dentine fail to mineralize but neither is peritubular dentine formed.

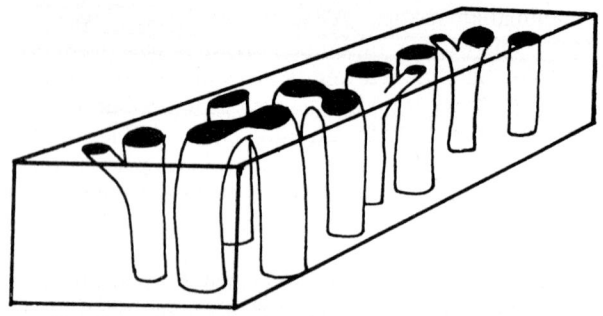

Fig. 52.—Tomes' granular layer may represent the cut ends of branching and bending tubules.

Within the subsurface of the root dentine is the 'granular layer of Tomes'. Since the last edition of this book an explanation for this anatomical feature has been proposed. Previously it was suggested that the granules consisted of minute interglobular spaces. However, the granules of Tomes' layer do not behave in the same way as interglobular dentine when viewed with either transmitted or incident light. The change in the optical properties of the granules of Tomes' layer when viewed first in transmitted and then in incident light indicates that the granules are true spaces. Yet when Tomes' granular layer is examined with the electron microscope no spaces are demonstrable. It has been suggested that the 'spaces' are produced by random looping of dentinal tubules (*Fig. 52*) in the first formed root dentine.

Outside Tomes' granular layer a thin (1 μm) structureless hyaline layer can frequently be seen in ground sections. The significance of this layer is not known but a number of recent studies suggests that it may be formed by the root sheath cells before they fragment and that this is the 'glue' which sticks cement to dentine.

Dentine formation continues slowly throughout life. The later formed dentine may be very difficult to distinguish from the first formed dentine, although it can often be recognized by a sudden change in the orientation of the tubules at the interface between the two. This later formed dentine is called 'physiological' (or 'regular') secondary dentine. At one time it was considered that this secondary dentine was formed beneath the cusps of teeth in response to attrition. However, this is unlikely to be true because it is formed in greater amounts at the floor of the pulp chambers in multi-rooted teeth, a position in which such a stimulus does not exist.

REFERENCES

Boyde A. and Lester K. S. (1966) An electron microscope study of fractured dentinal surfaces. *Calc. Tiss. Res.* **1**, 122.

Bradford E. W. (1967) Microanatomy and histochemistry of dentine. In: Miles A. E. W. (ed.), *Structural and Chemical Organization of Teeth*. New York, Academic.

Brannstrom M. and Garberoglio R. (1972) The dentinal tubules and the odontoblast processes. A scanning electron microscopic study. *Acta Odont. Scand.* **30**, 291.

Frank R. M. (1966) Étude au microscopie électronique de l'odontoblasts et du canalicule dentaire humaine. *Archs Oral Biol.* **11**, 179.

Johansen E. (1967) Ultrastructure of dentine. In: Miles A. E. W. (ed.), *Structural and Chemical Organization of Teeth*. New York, Academic.

Johansen E. and Parks H. F. (1962) Electron microscopic observations on sound human dentine. *Archs Oral Biol.* **7**, 185.

Kaye H. and Herold R. C. (1966) Structure of human dentine. 1, Phase contrast, polarization, interference and bright field microscopic observations on the lateral branch system. *Archs Oral Biol.* **11**, 355.

Kramer I. R. H. (1951) The distribution of collagen fibrils in the dentine matrix. *Br. Dent. J.* **91**, 1.

Lester K. S. and Boyde A. (1967) *See* Chapter 14.

Phillipas G. A. (1961) Influence of occlusal wear and age on formation of dentine and size of pulpchamber. *J. Dent. Res.* **40**, 1186.

Phillipas G. G. and Plebaurn E. A. (1966) Age factor in secondary dentine formation. *J. Dent. Res.* **45**, 778.

Schmidt H. (1961) Ein Beitrag zur Morphologie der Interglobularraume im verkalkten Dentin und ihr Nachweis der Entakalkung. *Archs Oral Biol.* **4**, 63.

Stahl S. S. and Slavkin H. C. (1972) Development of gingival crevicular epithelium and periodontal disease. In: Slavkin H. C. and Bavetta L. A. (ed.), *Developmental Aspects of Oral Biology*. New York, Academic.

Symons N. B. B. (1968) *Dentine and Pulp; A Symposium*. Edinburgh, Livingstone.

Ten Cate A. R. (1972) An analysis of Tomes' granular layer. *Anat. Rec.* **172**, 137.

CHAPTER 14

DENTINE SENSITIVITY

THE mechanism of dentine sensitivity is one of the most intriguing problems of dental histology and physiology. From common experience, most readers would not dispute that dentine is sensitive. This seems to imply the presence of nerve elements within the dentine but most of the nerve endings appear to be located within the pulp. It must also be remembered that histological studies alone cannot explain the mechanism of dentine sensitivity. All these can do is demonstrate a neuro-anatomical pathway associated with dentine sensitivity.

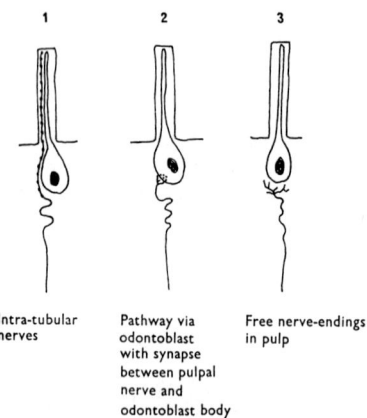

Fig. 53.—Diagram illustrating the possible neuro-anatomical pathways associated with dentine sensitivity.

Three possibilities exist which could explain the sensitivity of dentine. First, that the dentine is indeed innervated; second, that the odontoblast process and cell body have a special sensory function and are connected to a more normal neuro-anatomical pathway starting in the pulp; third, the receptors associated with dentine sensitivity are located within the pulp but are capable of detecting local changes conducted mechanically through the thickness of the dentine (*Fig. 53*). Each of these possibilities will now be discussed in turn, beginning with the evidence for the innervation of dentine.

No dispute exists about the presence of nerve trunks within the pulp. These can readily be demonstrated in several ways. Nor is there much dispute that these nerve trunks spread from the plexus of Raschkow beneath the odontoblasts (*Fig. 54*). The disputed point is whether or not finer nerve elements enter the dentine tubules and run as far as the enamel-dentine junction. Careful and controlled histological studies have shown that nerve-fibres leave the plexus of Raschkow, pass into the predentine as a loop, and pass out again to rejoin the plexus; also, what is more important, a few nerve fibres enter dentinal tubules. This has been demonstrated by light microscopy and confirmed by electron microscopy. However, considering the sensitivity of human dentine, remarkably few dentinal tubules appear to contain nerves, and, what is more significant, newly erupted teeth do not appear to contain intradentinal nerves despite the fact that they are sensitive.

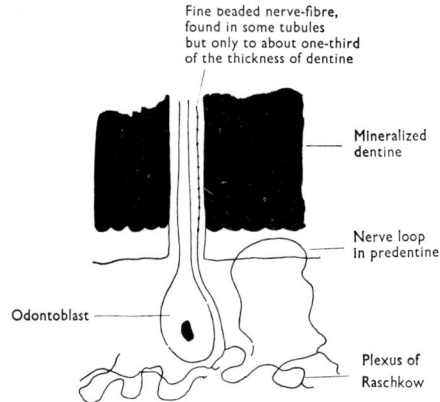

Fine beaded nerve-fibre, found in some tubules but only to about one-third of the thickness of dentine

Mineralized dentine

Nerve loop in predentine

Odontoblast

Plexus of Raschkow

Fig. 54.—Diagrammatic illustration of the location of nerves in dentine.

The few nerve fibres which enter dentinal tubules do not appear to penetrate far beyond the dentine/predentine junction. It might be argued that many nerves reach close to the enamel/dentine junction but that due to the difficulty in getting fixatives to penetrate dentinal tubules the deeply placed nerve fibres have degenerated and are therefore unrecognizable. The closer an intradentinal nerve is to the pulp of the tooth the better it will be fixed, and the more likely it is to be recognized in histological sections. However, the absence of any cytoplasm in the outer halves of dentinal tubules (*see* Chapter 13) indicates that this region does not contain nerves.

Those nerve fibres which do enter dentinal tubules are identified in electron microscope studies by the mitochondria and vesicles which they contain. Paradoxically, these features suggest, not that the nerve fibre is monitoring changes in its environment, but rather

91

that it is affecting the activity of the adjacent odontoblast process. This view, that the nerve fibres in dentinal tubules are motor rather than sensory nerves, receives support from the demonstration of adrenergic activity in the dentine. In other words, the nerves may be motor sympathetic terminals rather than sensory branchial receptors. However, the adrenergic activity of the dentine is not affected by cutting the cervical sympathetic chain. Had this operation abolished the adrenergic activity, it would have proved conclusively that the nerves in dentine were from the autonomic part of the nervous system. The problem remains to be solved. During the development of the tooth it is known that 'pioneer' nerve-fibres invade the dental papilla at the bell stage of development and that these fibres follow the path of the blood-vessels. However, the ramification of nerves which forms the plexus of Raschkow is not established until root formation is complete. This means that the nerve fibres must grow towards the dentine if its innervation is to be established (and/or secondary dentine encroaches on the pulp). The growing nerve tip approaching the predentine can find itself

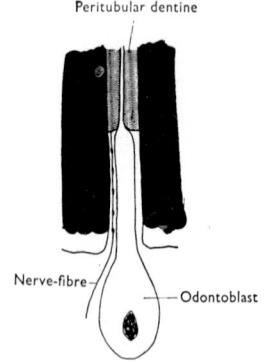

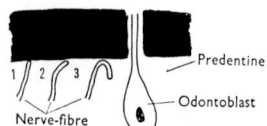

Fig. 56.—Diagram to illustrate three successive steps in the formation of a predentine nerve-loop.

Fig. 55.—Diagram showing how an intratubular nerve-fibre might be restricted by the peri-tubular dentine.

in one of two situations. It can by chance abut against the opening of the dentine tubule and pass into the lumen of the tubule, between the tubule wall and the odontoblast process. It is easy to conceive that such a growing tip pushes its way along the tubule until it meets the surface of the peritubular dentine when its extension ceases (*Fig. 55*). This would explain why intratubular nerve fibres are only found for a limited distance within the dentine and also why only a proportion of tubules contain them, their distribution depending on chance. The alternative situation is that a growing nerve fibre may not enter a dentine tubule but abut against the predentine surface. In this event, the growing tip will retract slightly and re-advance at a different angle. A succession of such steps would result in the looping of the nerve fibre (*Fig. 56*), and such loops could be caught up in the forming dentine.

It is thus fair to say that there is little doubt that mineralized dentine is innervated, but it is another question whether the presence of these few nerve fibres significantly influences the sensitivity of dentine. The histological demonstration of neural elements in dentine fails to explain the suggested hypersensitivity of the enamel-dentine junction or the sensitivity of newly erupted teeth.

We must now discuss the evidence for considering the odontoblast as a cell capable of transmitting a stimulus in a way that is comparable to a nerve. Such a hypothesis seems to require, first, that some form of impulse is propagated down an odontoblast, and, second, the presence of a functional connexion between the odontoblasts and those nerve-endings which continue to propagate the impulse. This functional connexion may or may not be a synapse.

In support of this it was at one time reported that acetylcholinesterase was present adjacent to the bodies and processes of the odontoblasts. This enzyme is typically found in association with nerves and its presence in dentine suggested an affinity between nerves and odontoblasts. Second, because odontoblasts are probably of neural crest origin it is not unreasonable to suggest that they may retain the ability of many neural crest cells (e.g. peripheral sensory nerves and postganglionic sympathetic nerves, whose cell bodies are outside the central nervous system) to propagate an impulse. Third, a recent electron-microscopic study has demonstrated what was described as 'a close functional relationship' (the term 'synapse' was specifically avoided) between nerve-endings and the processes of odontoblasts. Finally, the fact that odontoblast processes branch profusely in the region of the enamel-dentine junction could explain the reported hypersensitivity of the enamel-dentine junction on the basis of a summation phenomenon.

However, all the above findings have been either refuted or disputed. A more reliable method of assessing the presence of acetylcholinesterase has failed to demonstrate its presence in dentine. The membrane potential of odontoblasts has been measured in tissue culture (N.B., not *in vivo*) and found to be too low to take part in an excitable process. Substances known to cause pain when applied to bare nerve endings do not cause pain when applied to exposed dentine, while some substances which can cause pain when applied to dentine do not cause pain when applied to nerve endings. These findings all suggest that an odontoblast does not act as a type of nerve. As explained above, the close relationship between nerves and odontoblasts may be due to fortuitous growth rather than evidence of a functional relationship.

93

If the odontoblast process does not propagate an electrical impulse it remains to explain how a stimulus applied to the largely nerve-free dentine can be transmitted to the nerve endings deep within the tooth. The possibility exists of a purely physical rather than biological transmission of the stimulus. For example, it has been suggested that temperature changes at the surface of a tooth could be physically transmitted, by conduction, through the mineralized dentine to the pulp. But carefully timed responses to pain-producing stimuli have indicated that the speed of transmission is far greater than could be predicted by simple conduction. The times were closely related to those which could be predicted if the stimulus caused the movement of fluid through the dentine due to surface contractions and expansions consequent on temperature changes.

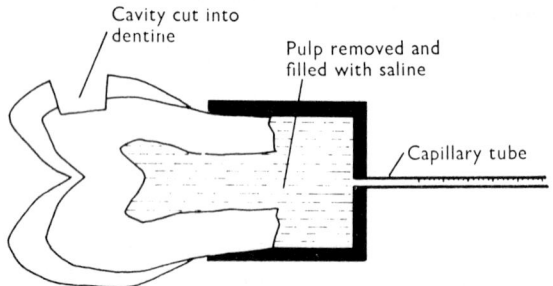

Cavity cut into dentine

Pulp removed and filled with saline

Capillary tube

Fig. 57.—Illustrating the method by which movements of fluid through dentine have been measured.

This is a part of the evidence which suggests that fluid movements in the dentine could be responsible for evoking the initiation of impulses from nerve-endings. It has not been found possible to test this directly; experiments have so far been limited to determining, first, whether fluid can move through dentine and, second, whether pain is evoked when the fluid can be presumed to have moved.

The rapid movement of fluid through dentine has now been demonstrated many times *in vitro*. A capillary is sealed to the root of a tooth from which the pulp has been removed (*Fig. 57*). The excavated pulp and the capillary are filled with saline. A cavity is cut into the dentine. If solutions of high osmotic pressure (for instance, sugar solutions) are applied to the cut surface of the dentine, fluid is rapidly sucked through the capillary. Still greater movements are produced by drying the dentine with a blast of air or by cutting the dentine with a drill.

It can be shown that each of the above operations causes pain *in vivo* and that the amount of pain is roughly proportional to the fluid movement observed *in vitro*. It is tentatively concluded that the movement of fluid through dentine causes stimulation of nerve endings either in the pulp or in the dentine. The fluid which moves may be accommodated in either the periodontoblastic space or the process of the odontoblast, or both. In any event, it is probably the eventual movement of interstitial fluid in the pulp which would initiate the stimulation of the nerve fibres. This is the basis of the suggestion that there is a hydrodynamic transmission of pain-producing stimuli.

Although the evidence for the concept that pulpal nerves originate the impulse has been summarized briefly here, sufficient has been written to indicate the present trend of opinion concerning dentine sensitivity. Some problems are still outstanding, mainly concerning the extracellular or intracellular nature of the fluid which may move in the dentine tubules. Furthermore, it is not known if the neural elements demonstrated in dentine can be totally excluded from the mechanism of dentine sensitivity.

If dentine is sensitive and pain is the only result of any successful stimulus, the painful sensation must have some selective advantage in terms of evolution. But it is remarkably difficult to conceive any advantage in this painful response. Potentially noxious excesses of temperature and pressure are monitored by the oral mucosa and periodontal ligament, tissues which are far more easily damaged than dentine. One possible answer is that when dentine has been worn away by attrition and there is no secondary dentine sealing the pulp, pain might be felt. This would encourage mastication of food in another part of the mouth until secondary dentine had been deposited.

Another solution to this problem suggests that dentine might act like an enormous pressure receptor, detecting the direction and amount of force applied to the individual cusps of teeth (nerves supplying the periodontal ligament can only integrate the direction and amount of force applied to every cusp on the tooth). When a cusp is compressed, fluid could be squeezed down dentinal tubules initiating a patterned response from the pulpal afferent nerve fibres which supply that cusp. This patterned response could be interpreted within the central nervous system as the direction and amount of pressure applied to a tooth cusp.

The above explanation needs to be compared with the generally accepted view that the movement of fluid down dentinal tubules evokes a sensation of pain in man (and all animals?). It is very unlikely that stimuli such as extremes of temperature, of dessication, and of osmosis are ever received by a normal dentition. The only naturally applied stimulus would be pressure. If pressure is applied to a tooth, it seems inevitable that periodontal afferents would be stimulated. Therefore, (almost) without exception, whenever fluid is moved down dentinal tubules by pressure applied to the cusp of a tooth (thereby stimulating pulpal afferents), periodontal afferents are simultaneously stimulated. In this situation, the discharge of pulpal afferents is not interpreted as pain. However, in an abnormal experimental situation it is possible to move large volumes of fluid down dentinal tubules (e.g. by applying solutions of high osmotic pressure) without stimulating periodontal afferents. Such large fluid movements would normally be associated with very heavy pressure on the tooth. In the absence of this expected sensation of pressure it is possible that the central nervous system interprets the abnormal isolated activity of pulpal afferents as a painful sensation.

REFERENCES

Anderson D. J. (1963) *Sensory Mechanisms in Dentine*. Oxford, Pergamon.

Anderson D. J., Hannam A. G. and Mathews B. (1970) Sensory mechanisms in mammalian teeth and their supporting structures. *Physiol. Rev.* **50**, 171.

Avery J. K., Cox C. and Corpron R. E. (1974) The effects of combined nerve resection and cavity preparation and restoration on response dentine formation in rabbit incisors. *Archs Oral Biol.* **19**, 539.

Bradlaw R. V. (1936) The innervation of teeth. *Proc. R. Soc. Med.* **29**, 507.

Brannstrom M. (1968) Physio-pathological aspects of dentinal and pulpal response to irritants. In: Symons N. B. B. (ed.), *Dentine and Pulp*. Edinburgh, Livingstone.

Brannstrom M. and Astrom A. (1972) The hydrodynamics of the dentine; its possible relationship to dentinal pain. *Int. Dent. J.* **22**, 219.

Fearnhead R. W. (1957) Histological evidence for the innervation of human dentine. *J. Anat., Lond.* **91**, 267.

Frank R. M. (1968) Relationship between the odontoblasts, its process and the nerve fibre. In: Symons N. B. B. (ed.), *Dentine and Pulp*. Edinburgh, Livingstone.

Powers M. M. (1952) The staining of nerve fibres in teeth. *J. Dent. Res.* **31**, 383.

Ten Cate A. R. and Shelton L. (1966) Cholinesterase activity in human teeth. *Archs Biol.* **11**, 423.

CHAPTER 15

AMELOGENESIS

ALTHOUGH enamel is ectodermal in origin, as opposed to mesodermal, and although it contains an extremely high proportion of inorganic salts (96 per cent by weight), its formation displays the same fundamental features found in the other mineralized tissues of the body; a cellular layer produces a matrix which is subsequently mineralized with hydroxyapatite.

At the bell stage of tooth development, when the crown pattern of the tooth is being determined, the base of the enamel organ consists of a single layer of short columnar cells, the internal enamel epithelium. The remaining tissues of the enamel organ are the stratum intermedium, stellate reticulum, and external enamel epithelium. At the time of differentiation of the odontoblasts, the cells of the

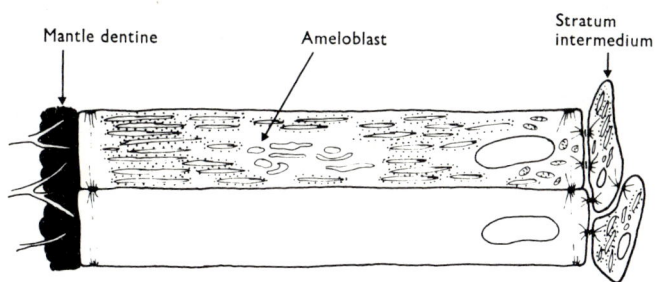

Fig. 58.—A newly differentiated ameloblast.

inner enamel epithelium increase in length, their cytoplasm accumulates an increasing amount of 'smooth' and 'rough' endoplasmic reticulum and free ribosomes, and their mitochondria move to the end of the cell nearest the stratum intermedium (*Fig. 58*). These changes are of a nature preparatory to the production of enamel; the cell is now termed an 'ameloblast'. The stratum intermedium and the inner enamel epithelium must be regarded as a single functional unit for the production of enamel. Alkaline phosphatase is found exclusively in the stratum intermedium during enamel matrix formation, while the internal epithelium is rich in RNA and has high oxidative enzyme activity. These histochemical features parallel those found in the cells forming other hard tissues.

The point has been made that the formative cells of the other hard tissues differentiate in regions of high vascularity. This is not so in the case of the cells of the internal enamel epithelium. These cells differentiate into functional ameloblasts in a relatively avascular situation. Not until the outer enamel epithelium becomes adjacent to the stratum intermedium with 'collapse' of the stellate reticulum does the former's rich capillary plexus provide the nutritive source for the ameloblasts. Until this vascular supply is established the ameloblasts are rich in glycogen and, because this is lost when the first increments of enamel matrix have been formed, the glycogen could be the source of energy used during the initial period of amelogenesis.

The onset of amelogenesis is marked by the aggregation of vesicles containing stippled material at the secretory pole of the ameloblasts. The vesicles fuse with the cell membranes and their contents become extracellular. This discharged material is the organic matrix of the first formed enamel. It is evident, therefore, that enamel is formed by a secretory process and not by conversion of the protoplasm of

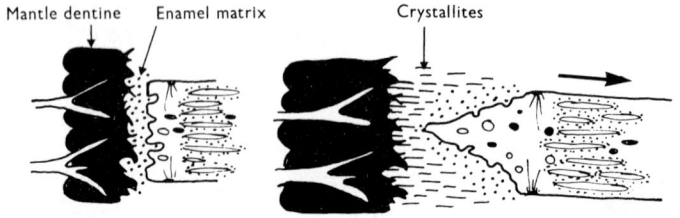

Fig. 59.—The start of enamel matrix formation and the development of a Tomes' process.

the ameloblast as was once believed. The ameloblasts move outwards away from the dentine surface as enamel matrix is secreted. When sufficient matrix has been deposited between the secretory end of an ameloblast and the outer surface of the dentine, the cell membrane of the ameloblasts becomes pushed into the matrix as the conical Tomes' process, through which further matrix is secreted (*Fig. 59*). The secretory activity of the ameloblast continues until the full enamel thickness is formed.

Unlike the other hard tissues there is no clear cut band of organic matrix such as predentine or osteoid preceding mineralization. Enamel crystallites appear almost immediately in newly secreted enamel matrix and by common usage the term 'enamel matrix' has come to be recognized as containing both organic and inorganic material. It seems likely that both the organic and the inorganic material are secreted together in the stippled vesicles (*see later*).

The nature of the organic component of enamel matrix is not yet fully understood. Apart from knowledge of the proportions of amino-acids there is as yet insufficient reliable knowledge of the structure of the proteins in enamel to present a 'textbook' description. The problem is largely related to the very small quantities of protein present in enamel and the difficulty of isolating it for analysis.

It is possible to demineralize enamel in several different ways to leave a 'soup' containing most of the organic material. There are probably several different proteins in enamel, each having a different solubility in differing demineralizing agents. During demineralization some of these proteins may become broken up into large polypeptides, some may remain unbroken. During the subsequent chemical procedures necessary to purify these proteins, other proteins may break up and some of the polypeptides may come together to form polypeptide aggregates of high molecular weight. These 'manufactured' aggregates may then be incorrectly identified as separate proteins. It is therefore very difficult to be certain, following a chemical analysis, that the resultant 'proteins' were in fact present in the original enamel.

Valuable information about the proteins can be indirectly obtained from analyses of the amino-acids. Thus it is possible to take the protein 'soup' referred to above, to break all the peptide bonds, and to analyse the proportions of the amino-acids present. The ratios referred to below were derived in this way. By comparing amino-acid analyses of developing and mature enamel it can be shown that large quantities of the amino-acid proline are removed during enamel maturation. This suggests that a protein (or it could be a polypeptide) which is rich in proline is selectively removed from enamel during enamel maturation.

It is thought by some that a keratin-like fibrous protein is present in the enamel matrix. The fibrous nature of this matrix seemed to be proved by the evidence of a complex of interlacing fibres seen with the electron microscope in carefully demineralized sections of enamel. Also various histochemical stains produced the same tinctorial picture in both enamel matrix and keratin. It has already been pointed out that the ultrastructure of the ameloblast does not conform to that of the keratinizing cell (Chapter 10). Electron microscopy of developing enamel and X-ray diffraction analyses of the unfixed matrix fail to reveal any evidence of a highly ordered fibre system. The similar staining reactions of enamel matrix and keratin can be explained when it is remembered that the stains employed demonstrate amino-acids and do not give any information as to how the amino-acids are assembled. In fact, biochemical analyses show that the ratios of amino-acids in forming enamel matrix are unique. Some salient features are an unusually high content of proline (25 per cent), the presence of the amino-acids histidine, lysine, and arginine in the ratio of 3 : 1 : 1, which is not comparable to the 1 : 4 : 12 ratio found in eukeratins and, lastly, the fact that cystine occurs in minimal amounts unlike the keratins which contain at least four times as much of this amino-acid (*Fig. 60*). The large number of proline residues in enamel matrix suggests the presence of a relatively unstable polypeptide. The protein molecules may be incorporated as a concentrated amorphous gel structure, rather than as an orientated assembly of fibres. It has also been suggested that this matrix has thixotropic qualities (ability to flow under pressure).

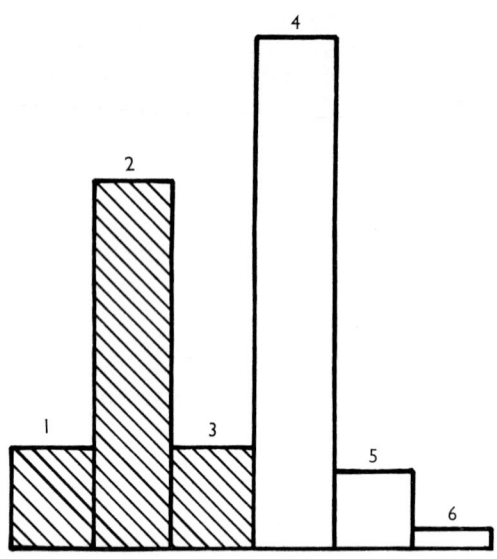

Fig. 60.—Histogram showing the change in amino-acid composition during enamel maturation. Cross hatched = before maturation. The numbers represent the number of amino-acid residues per 1000 total residues. 1, Glycine 67, 2, Proline 243. 3. Histidine 63. 4, Glycine 305. 5, Proline 47. 6, Histidine 9.

Support for these suggestions is gained from autoradiographic studies of sections of teeth of animals killed at various intervals after injection with labelled amino-acids. These studies demonstrate that although most incorporation of labelled amino-acids takes place rapidly into the newly formed enamel matrix, the labelled material subsequently spreads out, so that after several days all the formed matrix, i.e. matrix formed before and after injection, is labelled. This means that the proteins of the enamel matrix in which the amino-acids have been incorporated are labile. Within this distinctive matrix apatite crystals grow. Crystallites appear after the formation of a layer of enamel matrix about 50 nm thick: the initial epitactic foci may be the adjacent dentine hydroxyapatite. When they are first seen in the electron microscope the crystallites are thin and relatively widely separated within the matrix (*Fig. 61*). They thicken rapidly by addition to their sides and it is possible that the intervening matrix is squeezed out from between them in the direction of the ameloblasts where it might be utilized once more.

This mobility of enamel matrix may be of extreme importance in determining enamel structure and will be discussed at the conclusion of this chapter.

To obtain the final high degree of mineralization found in enamel fairly rapid changes occur in both the rate of mineralization and in the quality and quantity of the organic component of the matrix.

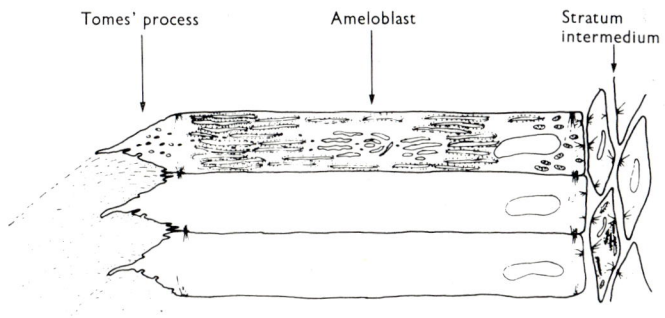

Fig. 61.—A fully differentiated ameloblast (seen in the longitudinal plane of a tooth).

There is a loss of water and amino-acids, especially histidine and proline, so that the final organic matrix of enamel not only has less protein but also is of different composition than that initially secreted by the ameloblasts. It now seems fairly certain that these changes in the organic matrix and the final influx of mineral salts involve activity of the ameloblasts. In the rodent incisor where the stages of enamel formation can be examined sequentially, it has been shown that the ameloblast at this time develops a brush border adjacent to the formed enamel matrix (in other words an increase in surface area) and that mitochondria accumulate adjacent to this brush border (*Fig. 62*). Activity of the enzyme acid phosphatase increases and amino-peptidase activity becomes demonstrable within the ameloblast for the first time. Both enzymes function in relation to catabolic events. For example, they are prominent in osteoclasts, cells associated with bone resorption, and it is not unreasonable to suppose that the ameloblasts are degrading material selectively removed from the enamel matrix. At the same time this cell is also

101

involved with the influx of mineral salts into the changing matrix. It has already been pointed out that during enamel matrix formation the mineral salts may be passed into the matrix via the secretory vesicles. This route is no longer available with the completion of matrix formation and the most likely way that mineral salts can now pass into enamel is across the brush border of the ameloblasts. There is evidence from other sources, such as calcium transport in the gut and in the avian shell gland, that activity of the enzyme alkaline phosphatase is required for calcium transport across membranes and it is perhaps significant that activity of this enzyme first occurs within the ameloblast at the time the brush border develops and indeed is associated with it. The ameloblast is capable, therefore, of secreting and removing material from enamel matrix during maturation of enamel. This ability to secrete and resorb material simultaneously may not be confined to the final stages of enamel maturation. There is fine structural evidence that the ameloblast may be doing just this throughout matrix formation with one surface of Tomes' process engaged in secretion and the other in absorption.

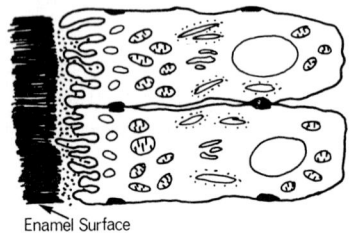

Enamel Surface

Fig. 62.—Ameloblasts at the end of amelogenesis: c.f. *Fig. 61.*

Reference has already been made to the fact that enamel formation occurs in two phases. First, a period where the entire thickness of enamel is laid down in the form of partially mineralized enamel matrix followed by a second phase of enamel maturation. This final mineralization occurs rapidly and enamel goes from a soft consistency to a very hard consistency in the time span of a few days. After this period of rapid mineralization it is sometimes assumed that the ameloblasts degenerate. However, the ameloblasts persist in a viable form up until the time of tooth eruption. There is evidence that during this time, that is between the completion of rapid enamel maturation and tooth eruption and which may be called the 'pre-eruptive maturation phase', important changes take place in the composition of enamel mediated by the ameloblasts. When enamel is analysed it is possible to show that gradients of concentration exist for several of its constituents. Thus the concentration of sodium, magnesium and carbonate is highest at the dentino–enamel junction and is almost halved in the surface layers of enamel. Conversely such elements as fluoride, lead, and zinc have their highest concentrations in the surface layers of enamel. These important gradients are established during the pre-eruptive phase of enamel maturation. Sodium, magnesium and carbonate, when incorporated into the hydroxyapatite crystal make it more soluble in water and acid. On the other hand fluoride, zinc, lead and tin, when combined with the hydroxyapatite crystal, make it less soluble in water and acid solutions. Thus these gradients have significance in terms of caries susceptibility as they all lessen the solubility of surface enamel. Furthermore, they are established during this pre-eruptive maturation phase as they can be demonstrated in the enamel of unerupted teeth.

These concepts of lability of the enamel matrix, simultaneous secretion and resorption by ameloblasts, together with the concept that the enamel crystallites may be aligned along lines of flow within the enamel matrix have been combined in a thesis which relates the development of enamel to its final structure. It must be emphasized that what follows is not proved experimentally (indeed it is difficult to see how it could be proved) and depends heavily on the use of analogues. Even so, because one of the aims of this book is to present current thought in each subject, no matter if later proved erroneous, we feel its presentation is justified.

As it is now generally agreed that enamel matrix is labile, flow lines must exist within it. How can it be demonstrated that crystallite orientation is related to these flow lines?

Two artificial systems have been designed to demonstrate this contention. The first is a smoke chamber in which convection currents are established in the smoke to mimic flow lines (*Fig. 63*). When these are observed through the glass plate forming the top of the smoke chamber, hexagonal patterns are seen which are similar to the cross-sectional appearance of the ameloblasts (*Fig. 64a*). If the glass plate is sheared, the hexagonal smoke patterns convert to a keyhole-shape resembling the cross-sectional appearance of human enamel prism (*Fig. 64b*). By moving the glass plate in different directions, smoke patterns conforming to the cross-sectional appearance of prisms in all types of enamel apart from that in rodents can be produced.

The second artificial system involves the use of iron filings and magnets. When magnets are drawn under a card sprinkled with iron filings, the filings arrange themselves along the lines of magnetic force. If the magnets are moved in a skewed manner so that a shearing component is introduced, the iron filings become orientated in such a way as to mimic the crystallite orientation seen in longitudinal sections of enamel. The results obtained from these two artificial systems suggest that the crystallites in enamel are orientated along lines of flow generated within the enamel matrix as it is secreted from the ameloblasts. The shearing factor is generated in human amelogenesis by virtue of the angulation of the ameloblast to the forming enamel front (*Fig. 65*).

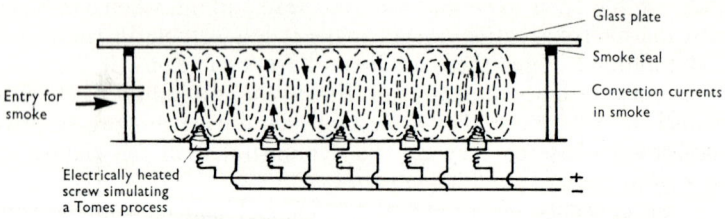

Fig. 63.—Diagrammatic section of the smoke chamber.

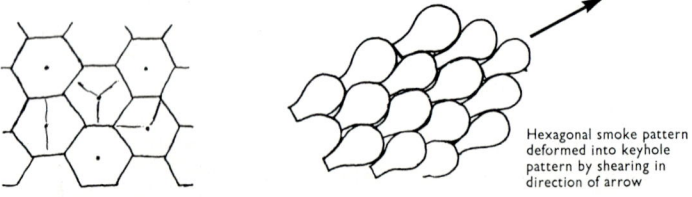

Fig. 64a.—Pattern seen in the smoke when viewed from above through the glass plate.

Fig. 64b.—Deformation of smoke pattern by moving glass plate in direction of the arrow.

Further possible support for the supposition that enamel crystallites orientation is related to flow may be derived from a study of the phylogeny of enamel. If reptilian enamel is examined, both fossil and modern, it is apparent that it has no prism structure and that its crystallites are arranged parallel to the long axes of the ameloblasts (*Fig. 67*). Furthermore, the reptilian tooth germ has little or no stellate reticulum. It has already been explained that the stellate reticulum is turgid (under pressure) in Chapter 5 and therefore must offer resistance to ameloblast movement. The implication is that in reptilian enamel development there is little resistance to ameloblast movement and that the crystallites will align along flow lines as depicted in *Fig. 67*. On the other hand, in modern mammals the development of the stellate reticulum, and with it the development of resistance to ameloblast movement, could result in the flow pattern illustrated in *Fig. 68*. In phylogenetic terms, therefore, it should be possible to predict that in fossil animals such as the mammal-like reptiles, enamel will have some form of intermediate crystallite orientation. A preliminary examination of fossil enamels has shown this to be the case and this provides evidence for the argument that the bulk of enamel structure is determined by crystallite orientation which is, in turn, determined by the flow patterns forming enamel matrix.

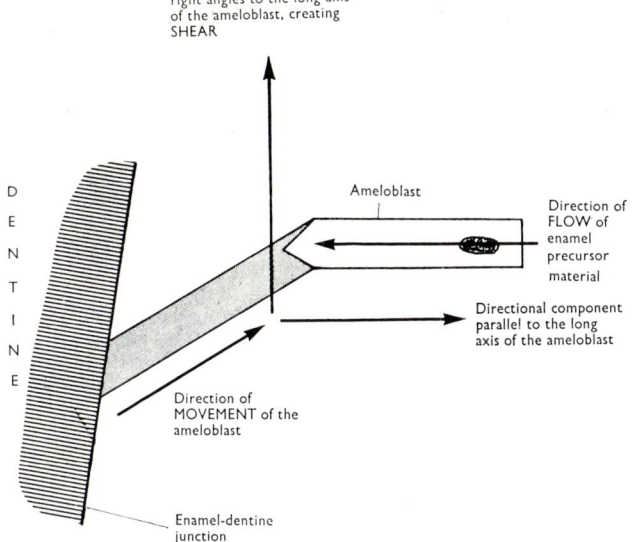

Fig. 65.—The direction of movement of an ameloblast can be resolved into two components, one at right angles to the long axis of the ameloblast and one parallel to the long axis. It can be seen that the former produces the shear.

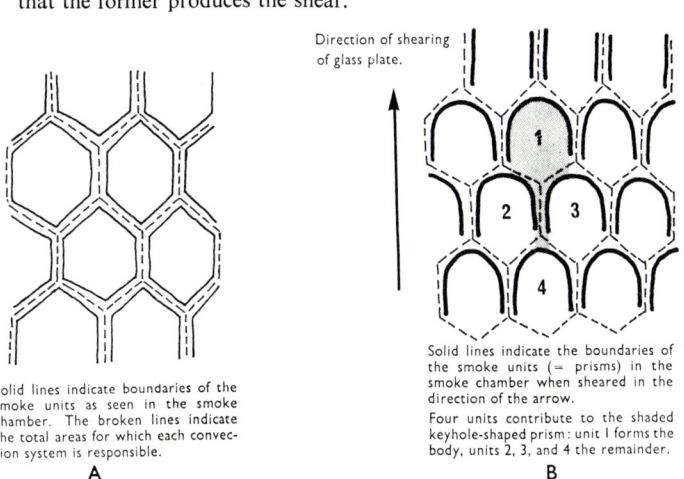

Solid lines indicate boundaries of the smoke units as seen in the smoke chamber. The broken lines indicate the total areas for which each convection system is responsible.

A

Solid lines indicate the boundaries of the smoke units (= prisms) in the smoke chamber when sheared in the direction of the arrow.

Four units contribute to the shaded keyhole-shaped prism: unit I forms the body, units 2, 3, and 4 the remainder.

B

Fig. 66.—Details of smoke patterns as seen from above. A, without shearing. B, when sheared.

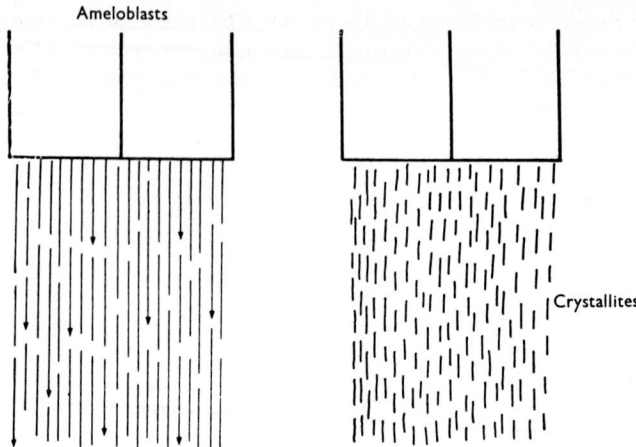

Fig. 67.—In reptiles, the small resistance to movement allows ameloblasts to move backwards rapidly. Flow lines in the secreted enamel matrix are parallel (left side) and therefore enamel crystallites are parallel to each other (right side) with the result that prisms are not formed.

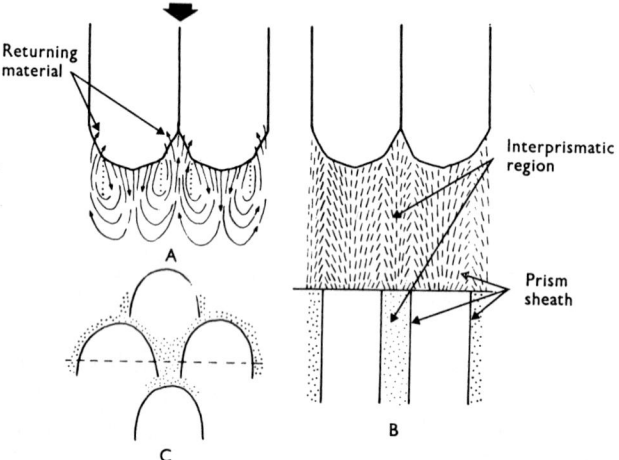

Fig. 68.—In mammals, the stellate reticulum and tooth follicle considerably restrain the backward movement of ameloblasts (A). The resulting compression of enamel matrix results in the flow lines shown in A. Crystals at the mineralizing front are orientated along these flow lines (B). The interprismatic region (stippled) develops opposite to those regions where material is being absorbed by ameloblasts. The prisms develop within newly secreted, as opposed to returning, material. The plane of section of B is illustrated in C. Note that this appearance, including the flattened Tomes' processes, is only seen in sections transverse to the long axis of a tooth (c.f. *Fig. 69*).

106

It will be noted from *Figs. 68* and *69* that prism bodies develop opposite secretory surfaces, the interprismatic region opposite absorbing surfaces and prism sheaths at the boundaries between secreting and absorbing surfaces. However, as with an equivalent line in the smoke chamber analogue (*Fig. 66b*), the predicted segment of prism sheath bounding the cervical edge of a prism disappears following shear (*Fig. 69*). By comparing *Figs 68* and *69* with *Fig. 66* it will be noted that each ameloblast forms one prism together with its surrounding interprismatic region.

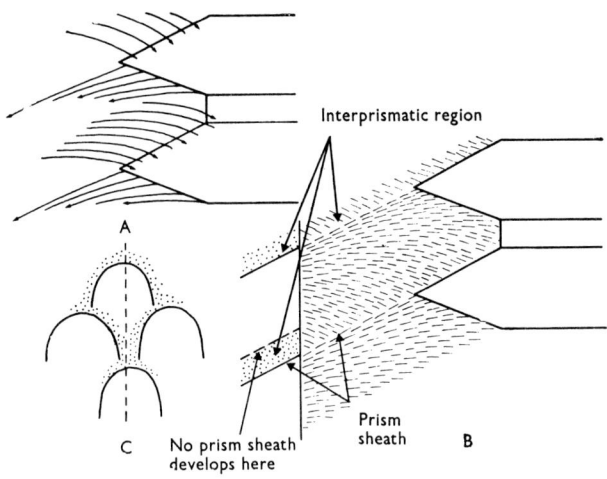

Fig. 69.—Amelogenesis seen in the longitudinal plane of a tooth. Just as in *Fig. 68*, prisms develop within newly secreted material and interprismatic regions in returning material. The altered flow (A) (c.f. *Figs. 63* and *68*) is due to shearing of the flow lines (*Fig. 65*). The plane of B is shown in C.

A recent electron microscope study of amelogenesis in the cat demonstrated a profound difference between the morphology of the cuspal and cervical surfaces of Tomes' processes. This lends support to the prediction implicit in *Fig. 69* that the cervical surface of a Tomes' process has a quite different activity (secretion) from that of the cuspal surface (absorption).

Finally, it begins to seem probable that most, if not all, of the material secreted by ameloblasts lies free within the cytoplasm of Tomes's processes rather than being contained in vesicles. This accords better with the flow concept outlined here. With this interpretation the stippled vesicles would contain absorbed material rather than secretion products.

REFERENCES

Burgess R. C. and Maclaren C. M. (1965) Proteins in developing bovine enamel. In: Stack M. V. and Fearnhead R. W. (eds), *Tooth Enamel I*. Bristol, Wright.

Crabb H. S. M. and Darling A. I. (1962) *The Pattern of Progressive Mineralization in Human Dental Enamel*. Oxford, Pergamon.

Deporter D. A. and Ten Cate A. R. (1975) Fine structural localisation of alkaline phosphatase in relation to enamel formation in the mouse molar. *Archs Oral Biol*. In the press.

Eastoe J. E. (1963) The amino-acid composition of proteins in dentine and enamel from developing human deciduous teeth. *Archs Oral Biol*. **8,** 633.

Kallenbach E. (1968) Fine structure of rat incisor ameloblasts during enamel maturation. *J. Ultrastruct. Res*. **22,** 90.

Kallenbach E. (1975) Fine structure of Tomes' process of the cat ameloblast. Abstract of a paper given at the 53rd Meeting of the International Association for Dental Research. *J. dent. Res*. Supplement.

Nylen M. U., Eames E. D. and Omnell K. A. (1963) Crystal growth in rat enamel. *J. Cell. Biol*. **18,** 109.

Osborn J. W. (1974) Variations in structure and development of enamel. In: Melcher A. H. and Zarb G. A. (ed), *Oral Sciences Reviews*, vol. 3. Copenhagen, Munksgaard, p. 3.

Reith E. J. (1970) The stages of amelogenesis as observed in molar teeth of young rats. *J. Ultrastruct. Res*. **30,** 111.

Ronnholm E. (1962a) The amelogenesis of human teeth as revealed by electron microscopy. II, The development of enamel crystallites. *J. Ultrastruct. Res*. **6,** 249.

Ronnholm E. (1962b) An electron microscopic study of amelogenesis in human teeth. I, The fine structure of ameloblasts. *J. Ultrastruct. Res*. **6,** 299.

Stack M. V. and Fearnhead H. W., ed. (1965) *Tooth Enamel I*. Bristol, Wright.

Young R. W. and Greulich R. C. (1963) Distinctive autoradiographic patterns of glycine incorporation in rat enamel and dentine matrices. *Archs Oral Biol*. **8,** 509.

CHAPTER 16

ENAMEL STRUCTURE

LIGHT microscopists had described all the known structures in human enamel, including the crystallites and their orientation (which had been inferred from polarization microscopy and X-ray diffraction studies), before the tissue was thoroughly investigated by electron microscopists. It is convenient to start with their observations because many of the structures they have described have yet to be seen by electron microscopists.

To the light microscopists the unit of enamel is the prism. It seems probable that most prisms extend through the full thickness of the enamel, widening from a diameter of about 3 μm near the enamel-dentine junction to about 6 μm at the surface of the tooth. This

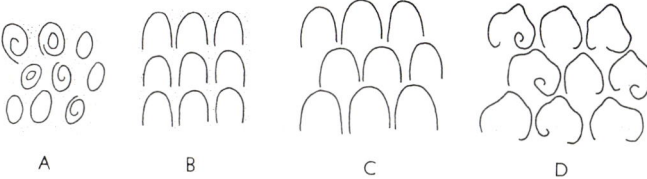

Fig. 70.—Illustrating the appearances of human enamel prisms in cross-section: A, Close to the enamel–dentine junction; B, At about 50μm from the enamel–dentine junction; C, Within most of the enamel; D, In some regions at the surface of the enamel. Generally agreed interprismatic regions are stippled.

widening is accounted for by the fact that near the enamel-dentine junction prisms are separated by larger interprismatic regions and also that the inner surface of the enamel has a smaller area than the outer surface. There is a little evidence that some prisms fail to reach the surface of the tooth from which it can be concluded that some ameloblasts might die before the full thickness of enamel is deposited.

Near the enamel–dentine junction, in true cross-section, human prisms may have any of the appearances shown in *Fig. 70A*. They are widely separated by an interprismatic region. At about 50 μm from the enamel–dentine junction they have enlarged considerably at the expense of the interprismatic region and are arranged as in *Fig. 70B*. At about 100 μm from the enamel–dentine junction they have the appearance shown in *Fig. 70C* and continue to appear like this until very close to the surface of the tooth, where they may again become very irregular (*Fig. 70D*) or their borders may disappear.

Within the past few years it has become fashionable to describe human enamel as consisting of 'keyhole-shaped' prisms (shaded in *Fig. 71B*), locked together in such a way that there is no interprismatic region. Previously the structure shown in *Fig. 71A* was described as consisting of roughly hexagonal or circular prisms separated by interprismatic 'substance', a material which was thought

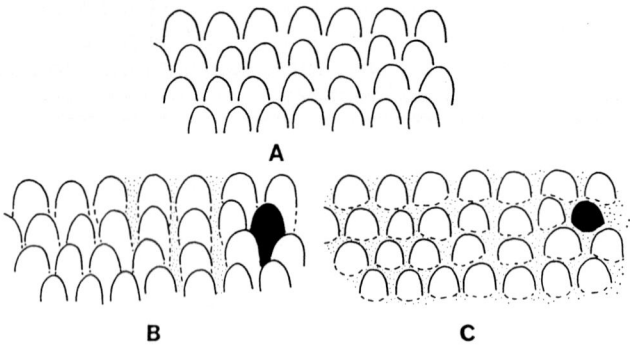

Fig. 71.—A, Typical appearance of human enamel prisms cut in cross-section. One terminology refers to the majority of these prisms as being 'keyhole-shaped' (black prism in B) and recognizes interprismatic regions only where they are stippled in this diagram. The other terminology (C) refers to prisms as 'roughly circular' (black) and to the remaining region as being 'interprismatic'.

to be less mineralized than the body of the prism (*Fig. 71C*). However, because electron microscopists have concluded that this latter 'substance' contains identical proportions of hydroxyapatite to that of the prism bodies it is preferable to use the term interprismatic 'region'. It will be observed from the diagram that the two conflicting descriptions of human enamel structure (keyhole-shaped prisms without interprismatic regions and circular prisms separated by interprismatic regions) are related solely to differences in terminology. There is no disagreement about the structure being described (*Fig. 71A*). Both interpretations require the construction of imaginary lines in order to complete the prism border. Because there is general agreement that all other forms of prismatic enamel contain interprismatic regions it seems to us that it is less confusing, more consistent, and probably more realistic to describe human enamel prisms as roughly circular, bearing in mind that the prism body is in continuity with the interprismatic region cervically.

Prisms bend from side to side in the transverse plane of the tooth but are approximately straight in the vertical plane of the tooth

110

(*Fig. 72*). A horizontal row of prisms all follow a similar path which is slightly out of phase with the paths of prisms in adjacent rows. This phase difference produces the sinuous structure shown on the left of *Fig. 72*. The sides of enamel crystals appear to reflect a small quantity of incident light. It can be seen that if incident light is reflected from the surface of a longitudinal section of enamel the shaded regions in *Fig. 72* would not reflect light up the microscope and would therefore appear dark. The unshaded regions would appear bright, because they reflect light up the microscope. This banded appearance is an epiphenomenon known as the 'Hunter-Schreger bands'. By changing the direction of the light the brightness of the bands is reversed. Towards the outer one-third of the enamel the prisms all pass straight to the surface and it is evident that it will no longer be possible to see bands.

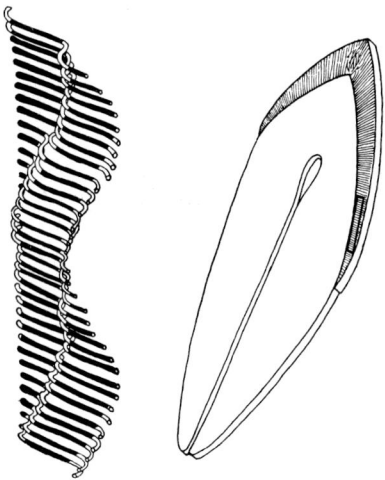

Fig. 72.—A ground section of a tooth is represented on the right. Prisms from the boxed region are represented on the left.

As a first approximation it is helpful to think of human enamel as consisting of a series of single-prism thick, coaxial, hollow cones with open apices lying against the enamel–dentine junction and their free edges at the surface of the tooth (*Fig. 73*). Each cone is a single layer of undulating tapered prisms. The phase difference between the bends of prisms contained in adjacent cones has been described above. At the tip of the cusp the apical angles of the cones are so acute that most longitudinal sections of a tooth cut the faces of several cones and the phase differences between the undulating prisms contained in each of the cones are superimposed on each other. The resultant apparent intertwining of prisms produces a gnarled appearance (gnarled enamel) which obscures a regularity of structure which can only be observed in transverse sections of the tooth taken through the cuspal enamel.

Contrary to previous descriptions, prisms in the cervical region of permanent teeth are not directed outwards and cervically but are generally approximately horizontal.

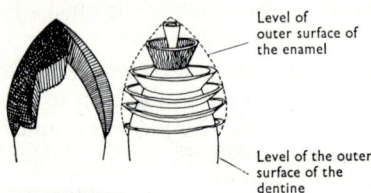

Level of outer surface of the enamel

Level of the outer surface of the dentine

Fig. 73.—Block diagrams illustrating the structure of enamel.

Three-dimensional reconstructions of enamel prisms reveal that many undulate at intervals of about 4–6 μm (*Fig. 74*). Previous studies of prisms seen in two dimensions suggested that these undulations were varicosities and constrictions. It has been speculated that these irregularities may correspond with the cross-striations of the prisms. This does not conflict with the speculation that the cross-striations may result from regular variations in the inorganic/organic ratio of substances along the length of the prism produced in response to a diurnal variation in the 4 μm per day rate of enamel formation.

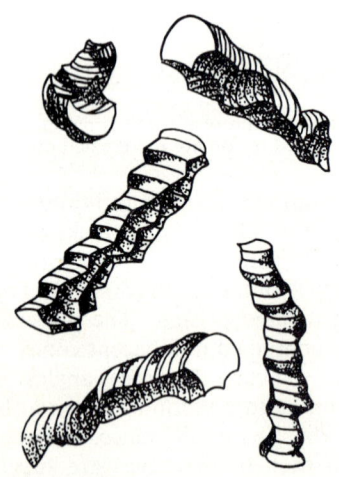

Fig. 74.—Drawings of wax-plate reconstructions of enamel prisms.

To the light microscopist the prism sheath appears to be about 0·5 μm wide. Apart from their observations on the structure of the interprismatic region, the other major contribution to an understanding of the morphology of enamel which has been contributed by electron microscopy is that the prism sheath is at most about 0·1 μm wide. A rapidly diminishing number of electron microscopists consider that a sheath *per se* does not exist and that a prism is bounded solely by an interface between crystallites of different orientation. However, a close study of electron micrographs which have been considered to demonstrate this interface seems always to reveal an irregular crystallite-free region (a region of microporosity) where the cervical ends of the crystallites in the more cuspal prism unevenly abut against the sides of the crystallites in the cervically adjacent prism (*Fig. 75*). Without the presence of this crystallite-free region (which, being unmineralized, has a refractive index quite different from that of the crystallites) it is difficult to explain why the sides of prisms reflect or scatter light in such a way that the sheath appears about 0·5 μm wide to the light microscopist. It has recently been shown that crystallites of the sheath region differ slightly in size from those of the prism.

Fig. 75.—Typical appearance of the border between two longitudinally sectioned prisms. There is a region of microporosity between the cervical border of the more cuspal prism and the cuspal border of the more cervical prism.

Within approximately 12 μm of the surface of the enamel, in many regions the crystallites are all parallel to the long axes of the prisms and the irregular, microporous, crystallite-free prism sheath no longer exists. The enamel in these regions therefore appears structureless to the light microscopist. The parallel arrangement (and therefore closer packing) of the crystallites and the absence of prism sheaths probably accounts for the observation that the surface enamel is the most highly mineralized.

The enamel surface of recently erupted and unerupted teeth has been studied by scanning electron microscopy. Although the majority of deciduous teeth contain regions in which the surface is structureless, such regions are far less common in permanent teeth. The perikymata (*see below*) crests may be structureless but prism outlines are nearly always visible in the troughs. These outlines often surround depressions about 2 μm deep which were, presumably, once occupied by the ageing ameloblasts. In some regions small hillocks of enamel up to 50 μm wide may project from the surface. The tops of these hillocks may be broken off to reveal irregular craters which have been called 'brochs'.

When sections of enamel are placed in aqueous solutions of certain substances some of the solution diffuses into the enamel and changes its optical properties, particularly the degree of birefringence. The change in birefringence can be measured and is related to the refractive index of the aqueous solution and the amount that diffuses into the enamel. Since the refractive index of the solution is known the amount that has diffused into the enamel can be calculated. It is found that the size of the molecules of the dissolved substance determine the amount which can penetrate into the spaces in the enamel and it is assumed that the volume diffusing when the solution of smallest molecular size is used represents the volume of spaces present in enamel. In this way it can be shown that enamel contains a system of micropores which act as a molecular sieve and that the volume of pores is about 0·2 per cent of the enamel volume. Attempts have been made to show that the optical properties of the striae of Retzius and the cross-striations are related to differences in the amounts of pores present in them as compared with the rest of the enamel.

The brown striae of Retzius seem to reflect a further phasic nature of enamel formation. The cross-striations are probably related to daily increments whereas the striae appear to be 4-day to 16-day increments.

It is generally supposed that, like the cross-striations, the striae are formed in relation to some systemic influence. Two features support this contention. First, neonatal lines seem to be well marked striae. Second, it has sometimes been observed that, taking into account the times at which they have been formed, the striae in all the teeth of a dentition are the same. In other words, the supposed systemic stimulus affected all developing teeth at the same time. However, so far the evidence for this later conclusion seems limited. In many sections of enamel striae are invisible because they are oblique to the plane of section; they can usually be seen if the section is tilted under the microscope.

It is a simple enough matter to observe brown striae but it has been found very difficult to give a uniform description of them. They may be between 150 μm thick down to the thickness of a cross-striation, they may be hypo or hypermineralized, they may be continuous or discontinuous, and clear striae, as opposed to brown, have also been described. The borders of prisms within the thicker brown striae are particularly optically dense and it may be that the brown colour is due to blue light (short wavelength) being abnormally scattered at these borders. This is supported by the observation that striae are blue-white when seen by reflected light. It has been speculated without evidence that within striae crystallites may be larger or smaller and that they may be orientated differently from crystallites in adjacent regions (similar speculations have been made on enamel structure in the region of the cross-striations).

It has been reported that in association with striae prisms may bend cervically or that they may bend in the transverse plane of the tooth.

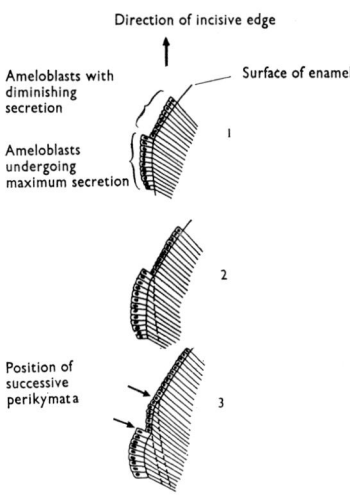

Direction of incisive edge

Ameloblasts with diminishing secretion

Surface of enamel

Ameloblasts undergoing maximum secretion

1

2

Position of successive perikymata

3

Fig. 76.—Diagrams of successive steps in the formation of perikymata, also showing their relationships to the brown striae of Retzius (broken lines).

If this latter observation is true, prisms have three 'curvatures'. A primary curvature (c.f. dentinal tubules) is responsible for the Hunter-Schreger band appearance and has a periodicity of about 1000 μm. A secondary curvature with a periodicity which may be from about 100 μm to about 16 μm is related to the striae of Retzius. A tertiary curvature, or undulation, with a periodicity of 4 μm is related to the cross–striations.

A series of fine furrows and ridges can be seen surrounding the surface of young teeth. These are called 'perikymata'. Ground longitudinal sections of teeth show that the brown striae meet the enamel surface at the furrows. From this relationship it is suggested that, during amelogenesis, a certain number of ameloblasts cease secreting at the same time. The series of ameloblasts immediately basal to these continue to secrete and the repetition of this cycle produces the system of perikymata (*Fig. 76*). The scanning electron microscope has shown that in the base of the furrows prism outlines can be distinguished.

115

Three further features of enamel can be seen in ground sections. Enamel lamellae are irregular vertical sheets of organic or hypo-mineralized matrix extending from the tooth surface often as far as, and occasionally beyond, the enamel–dentine junction. It has been suggested that they develop along planes of tension within the developing enamel, a slight disturbance leading to a failure of mineralization along the plane. Some of these lamellae may open up during development and cells from the enamel organ collect in the cleft. Finally, with advancing age, a third type of lamella may form in which the underlying dentine tends to contract so that the enamel, now unsupported, fractures. Organic material from the oral cavity will then collect in the split.

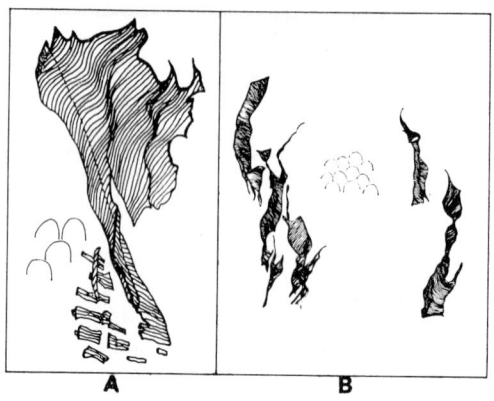

Fig. 77.—Reconstruction of tufts in enamel. The enamel cusp is towards the top and the cervical margin towards the bottom. The prisms outlines indicated in each reconstruction are about 5μm wide.

Groups of ribbon-like structures extend from the enamel–dentine junction into the enamel for up to one-third of its thickness. These constitute the 'enamel tufts', so called on account of their resemblance, when seen in transverse ground sections of teeth, to tufts of grass. A reconstruction of a small part of a tuft is shown in *Fig. 77*. Each tuft consists of a number of disconnected 'leaves' which appear to coincide with thickenings of the prism sheaths. In a recent study it was pointed out that when a substance changes from the liquid to the solid state contractions occur. In enamel, hydroxyapatite changes from the ionic (liquid) state in the ameloblast secretions to the solid state in the enamel crystallites. With the change of state, contractions will be expected and it is possible that these contractions could lead to the widening of prism sheaths which corresponds with the tufts. Evidently the tufts will follow the direction of prisms.

Microradiographic techniques show these regions to be hypocalcified, while diffusion experiments show them to be more permeable.

Frequently one can find in ground sections evidence of the continuation of dentinal tubules across the enamel–dentine junction into the enamel. These constitute the enamel spindles and they are to be found beneath the tips of cusps. The spindles lie parallel to the long axes of the ameloblasts at the start of amelogenesis and they become partly mineralized along with the developing enamel.

REFERENCES

Boyde A. (1969) Electron microscopic observations relating to the nature and development of prism decussation in mammalian dental enamel. *Bull. Group int. Rech. scient. Stomat.* **12,** 151.

Fosse G. (1964) The number of prism bases on the inner and outer surface of the enamel mantle of human teeth. *J. Dent. Res.* **43,** 57.

Fosse G. (1968) A quantitative analysis of the numerical density and the distributional pattern of prisms and ameloblasts in dental enamel and tooth germs. *Acta Odont. Scand.* **26,** 573.

Fujita T. (1939) Uber die Retzius' schen Parallelstreifen des Zahnschmelzes. *Anat. Anz.* **86,** 350.

Glas J. E. and Nylen M. U. (1965) A correlated electron microscopical and microradiographic study of human enamel. *Archs Oral Biol.* **10,** 893.

Gustafson A. (1959) A morphologic investigation of certain variations in the structure and mineralization of human dental enamel. *Odont. Tidskr.* **67,** 361.

Gustafson G. and Gustafson A. (1967) Microanatomy and histochemistry of enamel. In: Miles A. E. W. (ed.), *Structural and Chemical Organization of Teeth*, vol 2. New York, Academic.

Gustavsen F. and Silness J. (1969) Crystal shape in the prism sheath region of sound human enamel. *Acta Odont. Scand.* **27,** 617.

Helmcke j.-G. (1967) Ultrastructure of enamel. In: Miles A. E. W. (ed.), *Structural and Chemical Organization of Teeth.* New York, Academic.

Heuser H. (1961) Die struktur des menslichen zahnschmelzes in oberflach en histologischen bild (replica technik). *Archs Oral Biol.* **4,** 50.

Johnson N. W. (1967) Some aspects of the ultrastructure of early human enamel caries seen with the electron microscope. *Archs Oral Biol.* **12,** 1505.

Meckel A. H., Griebstein W. J. and Neal R. J. (1965) Structure of mature human dental enamel as observed by electron microscopy. *Archs Oral Biol.* **10,** 775.

Osborn J. W. (1965) The nature of the Hunter-Schreger bands in enamel. *Archs. Oral Biol.* **10,** 929.

Osborn J. W. (1974) Variations in the structure and development of enamel. In: Belcher, A. H. and Zarb G. A. (ed.), *Oral Sciences Reviews*, vol. 3. Copenhagen, Munksgaard, p. 3.

Poole D. F. G. and Brooks A. W. (1961) The arrangement of crystallites in enamel prisms. In: Belcher, A. H. and Zarb G. A. (ed.), *Oral Sciences Reviews*, vol. 5. Copenhagen, Munksgaard, p. 14.

Ripa L. W., Gwinnett A. J. and Buonocore M. G. (1965) The prismless outer layer of deciduous and permanent enamel. In: Belcher A. H. and Zarb, G. A. (ed.), *Oral Sciences Reviews*, vol. 5. Copenhagen, Munksgaard, p. 41.

Schour I. and Hoffman M. M. (1939) Studies in tooth development II. The rate of apposition of enamel and dentine in man and other mammals. *J. Dent. Res.* **18**, 161.

Stack M. V. and Fearnhead R. W., ed. (1965) *Tooth Enamel.* Bristol, Wright.

CHAPTER 17

CEMENTOGENESIS

CEMENTOGENESIS begins shortly after the fragmentation of Hertwig's root sheath. Fragmentation of the root sheath permits penetration of the connective tissue cells of the follicle so that they come to lie between the remnants of the root sheath and the surface of the newly formed root. There is now an increasing amount of evidence to suggest that the surface of the newly formed root is covered by an epithelial product formed by the epithelial cells of Hertwig's root sheath before they fragment. This layer is approximately 1 μm thick, appears hyaline in the light microscope and as a granular layer containing a few fine collagen fibres in the electron microscope. Significantly, as this layer forms the root sheath cells develop increasing amounts of rough endoplasmic reticulum indicative of secretory activity. Biochemical analysis indicates the presence of both collagen and epithelial derived amino-acids. The ability of dental epithelium to produce collagen has already been indicated.

The ectomesenchymal cells (*see* Chapter 19) of the follicle after penetrating the root sheath differentiate into cement-forming cells or cementoblasts. The cells are characterized by the presence of numerous mitochondria, a great deal of rough surfaced endoplasmic reticulum, and a prominent Golgi complex. Histochemically they have a high hydrolytic and oxidative enzyme content. There is evidence that at the time of disruption of Hertwig's sheath, there is a local increase in the number of collagen fibres of the follicle, so that the connective tissue which ultimately intervenes between the root sheath and the dentine is predominantly fibrous. The factors responsible for cementoblast differentiation and for the increased fibrillogenesis are unknown.

The fibrous connective tissue in contact with the surface of the root contributes to the first formed cement matrix. It would appear, however, that additional collagen fibres and ground substance are contributed as a result of cementoblast activity to form the definitive unmineralized cement matrix or cementoid (*Fig. 78*). The formation of cement matrix has therefore many parallels with the formation of the dentine matrix in that in both cases there is a dual origin of fibres and of ground substance. When sufficient organic matrix has been formed it becomes mineralized by the deposition within it of hydroxyapatite in the form of either plates or spicules. The manner in which the crystallites are deposited within the cement matrix

119

has recently been investigated and found to occur as follows. They form at the dentine cement interface, growing from the crystals of the dentine (or of the hyaline layer) into, onto and between the collagenous fibrils of the cement matrix.

As matrix formation proceeds, the cement-forming cells can be incorporated within the developing cement where they become cementocytes, or they may remain on the surface of the forming cement as more rounded cells lacking processes. Two types of cement are thus recognized, cellular and acellular respectively. Cementocytes are characterized by processes radiating towards the periodontal ligament and their cytoplasm shows a drastic reduction in the number of organelles when compared to the cementoblast (*Fig. 31*).

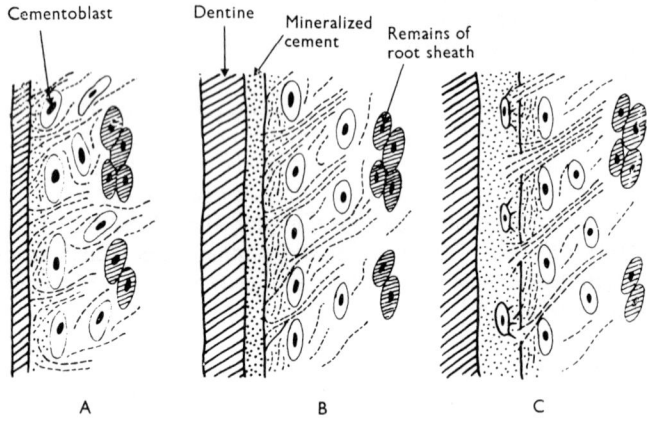

Fig. 78.—The matrix of the earliest formed cement is almost all contributed by the periodontal ligament rather than by cemento-blasts (A). In later formed cement, (B) and (C), progressively more matrix may be secreted by cementoblasts. The cores of the Sharpey fibres may not mineralize (C).

As well as distinguishing two types of cement on the basis of their cellular content it is also possible to distinguish differences between their organic matrices.

Cement is the tissue whereby the fibres of the periodontal ligament gain attachment to the root of the tooth. Before the tooth erupts the fibres of the tooth follicle become incorporated in the cement matrix. These original fibres are arranged approximately parallel to the root surface. After eruption of the tooth, however, the fibres of the periodontal ligament lie oblique to the root surface and it is obvious that they must be incorporated within the cement, otherwise

no attachment would be made. These principal fibres of the periodontal ligament are large, rope-like bundles of collagen fibres which
as they approach the cement, untwine to form smaller fibre bundles.
The bulk of the collagen fibres in acellular cement are formed from
these ligament fibre bundles (Sharpey fibres) (*Fig. 78A*). Once incorporated within the acellular cement they become fully mineralized
and indistinguishable from the few other fibres of the cement matrix.
This type of cement, therefore, most likely serves the purpose of
anchoring the tooth in the alveolus and explains why it is found
applied to the coronal two-thirds of the root. On the other hand,
cellular cement has only some 40–60 per cent of its collagen content
derived from Sharpey fibres (*Fig. 78B*). The remainder are intrinsic
fibres. Many of the Sharpey fibres passing into cellular cementum
only mineralize at their periphery and thus have an unmineralized
core (*Fig. 31*).

It has recently been suggested that the time-honoured classification
of cement into cellular and acellular types is too trivial in terms of
development and structure. It may be more useful to think in terms
of 'predominant' Sharpey fibre cement (*Fig. 78A*) and 'partial'
Sharpey fibre cement (*Fig. 78C*). The first formed cement is 'predominant' Sharpey fibre and does not contain cells. The later
formed cement is 'partial' Sharpey fibre and although it usually
contains cells it can sometimes be acellular.

In general there is a direct relationship between the thickness of
cement and the age of the tooth. However, its growth is most rapid
in the apical regions where it is formed to compensate for active
eruption of the tooth which itself compensates for occlusal wear.
The phasic nature of its deposition results in incremental lines which
have been described as hyper- or hypomineralized. No explanation
has been offered for the presence of hypermineralized lines but the
hypomineralized lines are comparable to the resting lines present in
bone.

On the surface of the root dentine in premolars and molars a
variety of cement characterized by wide irregular branching spaces
is frequently found. This is the intermediate cement. There is a
disagreement as to the origin of the cells that at one time occupied
these spaces. It has been suggested that these spaces once contained
epithelial cells derived from Hertwig's root sheath that had become
trapped on the dentine surface during the formation of the first
layers of dentine. Alternatively, that during eruption of the cheek
teeth cementocytes, whose processes have become attached to the
cement and whose periodontal surface is attached to the connective
tissue, become pulled upwards and distorted by movement of the
erupting tooth. A further opinion asserts that the lacunae in this
type of cement are occupied by odontoblasts which are trapped on

121

the outer surface of the dentine at the start of dentinogenesis, subsequently being engulfed by the forming cement. The many interpretations of intermediate cement may be the result of species differences. It has recently been shown that in the rodent epithelial root-sheath cells do become trapped in first formed cement. However, several studies on cementogenesis provide no evidence of entrapment of root-sheath in man. On the other hand, human intermediate cement has been shown to contain cells, larger than cementocytes, which are surrounded by unmineralized areas. The origin of these cells remains speculative but it seems that a root sheath origin can be excluded.

REFERENCES

Bernard G. W. (1970) Initial calcification of cementum. Abstract of a paper given at the 48th meeting of the International Association for Dental Research. *J. Dent. Res.* Supplement.

Boyde A. and Jones S. J. (1972) Scanning electron microscope studies of the formation of mineralised tissues. In: Slavkin H. C. and Bavetta L. A. (ed.), *Developmental Aspects of Oral Biology*. London, Academic, p. 243.

Furseth R. (1969) The five structures of the cellular cementum of young human teeth. *Archs Oral Biol.* **14,** 1147.

Lester K. (1969) The incorporation of epithelial cells by cementum. *J. Ultrastruct. Res.* **27,** 63.

Listgartern M. A. (1970) Ultrastructure of cementogenesis in human teeth. Abstract of a paper given at the 48th meeting of the International Association for Dental Research. *J. Dent. Res.* Supplement.

Owens P. D. A. (1972) Light microscope observations on the formation of the layer of Hopewell-Smith in human teeth. *Archs Oral Biol.* **17,** 1985.

Selvig K. A. (1964) Ultrastructural study of cementum formation. *Acta Odont. Scand.* **22,** 105.

CHAPTER 18

ROOT FORMATION

IT will be recalled from reading Chapter 3 that the outer and inner enamel epithelia are continuous at the cervical edge of the enamel organ, forming the cervical loop. In the late bell stage of development, when apposition of the hard tissues of the crown is well advanced, the cervical loop grows to form a double layer of epithelial cells known as 'Hertwig's root sheath'. It is under the influence of this sheath that the roots develop. Frequently one finds in histological sections a few stellate cells sandwiched between the inner and outer epithelia in the root sheath. During development, Hertwig's sheath grows basally between the tooth follicle and the dental papilla and it comes to enclose the papilla except for an opening at its base, known as the 'primary apical foramen' (*Fig. 79*). Hence, root morphogenesis is bound up with the dynamic activity of Hertwig's sheath.

At first Hertwig's sheath is angled beneath the dental papilla in which form it has been termed a 'root diaphragm'. It seems likely that the base of the growing dental papilla pushes the root sheath outwards moulding it to the shape of the base of the fibrous follicle. As the major cusps form on the crown of a molariform tooth, the papilla pushes irregularly outwards as a number of lobes. These lobes produce corresponding 'bays' in the outline of the root which surrounds it. The 'bays' correspond in number and location with the definitive roots (*Fig. 80*). The tongues of epithelial tissue separating the bays now grow inwards to outline the secondary apical foramina and to fuse near the centre of the crown base: the number of the roots thus corresponds with the number of bays in the root diaphragm. The fact that the outward expansion of the papilla generates bays in the root diaphragm might create the impression that there is no intrinsic growth in the diaphragm. However, although not as abundant as might be expected, mitosis figures are found in the cells of the diaphragm from its inception indicating its growth in area. This growth is masked because the base of the dental papilla is expanding at the same rate as the root diaphragm is growing to surround it. Only in regions where the rate of ectodermal growth is greater than the rate of expansion of the base of the dental papilla can the ectoderm divide the root base into separate root areas.

Each secondary apical foramen will ultimately open at a root apex. Where the tongues of tissue meet, running from near the centre of the crown base to the inner aspect of each root, junction lines form, which may be visible as low dentine ridges on the completed tooth. Local defects may occur along these junction lines to produce pulpo-periodontal canals each containing a blood-vessel and a nerve. These are found most commonly in the root bifurcations of deciduous molars. If the adjacent sheaths remain slightly separated in the region of the junction narrow dentine bridges connecting adjacent roots may be formed.

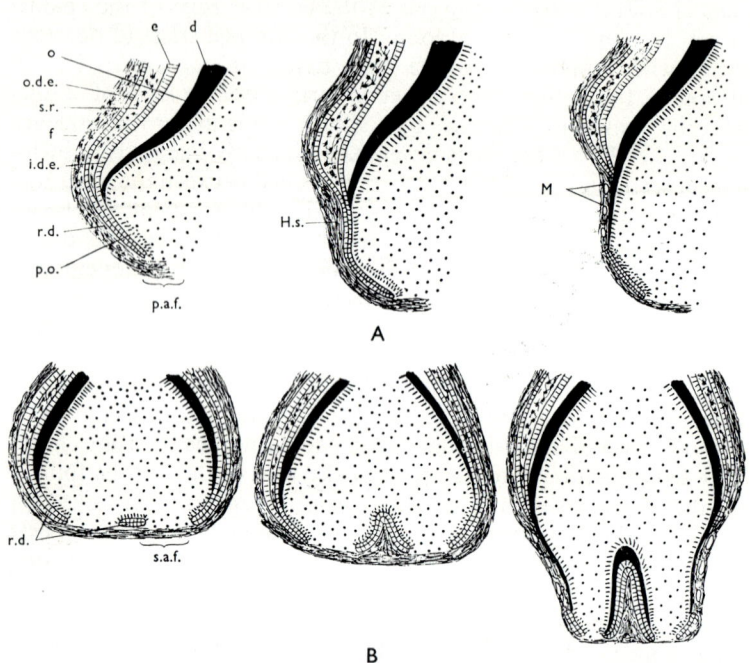

Fig. 79.—Diagrams of three successive stages in root formation, A, in a single-rooted tooth, B, in a two-rooted tooth. Not to scale. d, dentine; e, enamel; f, tooth follicle; H.s., Hertwig's root sheath; i.d.e., inner dental epithelium; M, Malassez rests; o, odontoblasts; o.d.e., outer dental epithelium; p.a.f., primary apical foramen; p.o., differentiating odontoblasts; r.d., epithelial root diaphragm; s.a.f., secondary apical foramen; s.r., stellate reticulum. In A there is a single persistent primary apical foramen. In B the primary apical foramen is rapidly divided to produce two secondary apical foramina.

It will be recalled that when discussing the blood-supply to the tooth it was shown that vessels entering the dental papilla collect in groups whose number and disposition predict the location of the definitive roots. These groups of vessels lie in the bays in the developing root diaphragm, and the tissue tongues expand inwards between the vessels to unite in the less vascular centre of the crown base.

In single rooted teeth the procedure is precisely the same but no bays form in the free edge of the root diaphragm, probably due to the absence of developing lobes in the dental papilla. Furthermore, pulpo-periodontal canals are less common in the coronal half of these teeth.

Once the secondary apical foramina have been delineated in a multi-rooted tooth, a true Hertwig's sheath is present. This continues to grow in a vertical direction. The length of the root is a function of either the degree of intrinsic growth of Hertwig's sheath or of growth of the dental papilla and it is not yet conclusively established which tissue plays the dominant role.

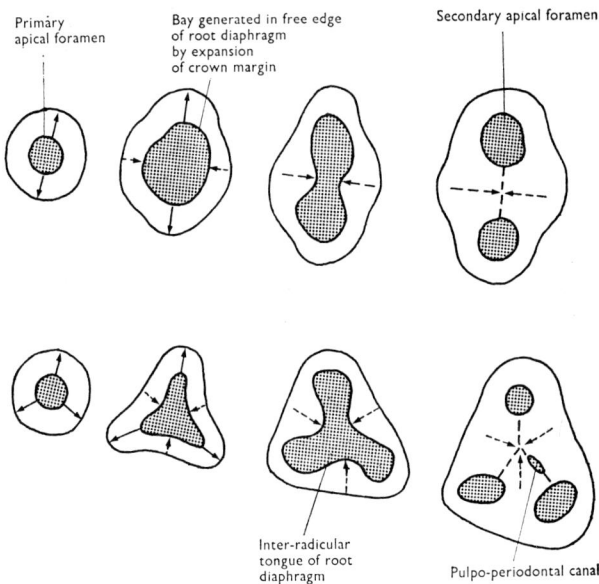

Fig. 80—Diagrams showing successive stages in the process of subdivision of the primary apical foramen; as seen from below, producing a two- and a three-rooted tooth. The shaded area represents the papilla seen through the apical foramen. The solid arrows show the direction of expansion of the crown margin. The broken arrows show the direction of growth of the inter-radicular tissue tongues of the root diaphragm. Not to scale.

As Hertwig's sheath grows vertically, it induces the differentiation of odontoblasts at the papilla surface. The odontoblasts produce the dentine of the root which lengthens in an apical direction.

After completing its organizing function, Hertwig's sheath fragments, remnants persisting in the adult periodontal ligament as the epithelial cell rests of Malassez. Various functions have been

125

ascribed to these cell rests from time to time, though without any evidence. Histochemical studies reveal the continuing viability of these cells throughout life, albeit in a quiescent state so that the term 'rests' is a reflection of their metabolic state. The following suggestion is offered to explain the fragmentation of Hertwig's root sheath. It was noted that during the formation of the bud, cap, and bell stages of tooth development the free margin of the enamel organ (the cervical loop) grows around the expanding dental papilla. It has been demonstrated by serial radiographic examination that the tip of a growing root does not penetrate far into the basally adjacent alveolar bone until the tooth has erupted into the oral cavity and met its opponent (*Fig. 81*). Because the tip of the growing root is roughly stationary then so also is the tip of Hertwig's root sheath.

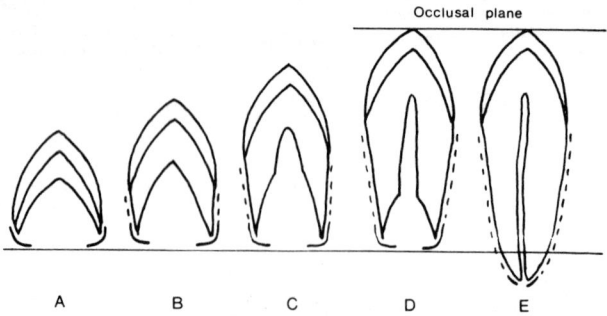

Fig. 81.—Four stages in the development and eruption of a tooth. During stages A, B, and C the tip of the lengthening root is maintained at the same distance from the lower border of the mandible. Alveolar bone develops around the erupting tooth. While the tooth erupts Hertwig's root sheath is pulled coronally together with the moving root. When the crown meets the opposing tooth the root begins to extend back into the jaw.

In other words Hertwig's root sheath is not growing downwards into the jaw but the root dentine (and enamel) are moving away from it (*Fig. 81A–D*). As the cells of the root sheath proliferate in their continuing attempt to surround the dental papilla they may be pulled towards the oral cavity by the moving root. Because it is being pulled coronally by the lengthening root the proliferating root sheath is prevented from growing round the base of the papilla and sealing the apical foramen. The pull produces tension on the sheet of epithelial cells splitting it into a fenestrated pattern. This may explain why no degeneration of root-sheath is seen when it breaks up. When the erupting tooth has met its opponent the lengthening root can no longer slide past the root sheath which will now start to encircle the base of the papilla and complete the formation of the apical foramen of the tooth (*Fig. 81E*).

Although in Hertwig's sheath the cell layer nearest the papilla is directly continuous with the inner enamel epithelium over the crown, its cells do not pass through the same cycle of histodifferentiation, nor do they normally produce any enamel. The histochemical content of the two cell strata is different. Commonly, however, small enamel pearls are formed on the surface of roots, particularly at the bifurcation of roots. This shows, therefore, that some root-sheath cells are potentially capable of producing enamel. It is well known that coronal odontoblasts differentiate under the influence of the overlying inner enamel epithelium. There is no doubt that a similar inductive function is the prime role of Hertwig's sheath.

Unsuccessful attempts have been made to correlate the number and location of the roots with the position of the major cusps on the crown of the molariform tooth. In the late 18th century it was suggested that a relationship existed between the pattern of blood-vessels supplying the developing tooth and the presence of morpho-genetic fields within it. More recently, these fields have been equated with cuspal areas, thought to be controlled by growth centres located within the pulp, under the influence of which specific parts of the crown pattern are generated. Direct evidence of these areas and centres is lacking, but it seems reasonable to expect that each should receive an adequate blood-supply via the roots. Hence the number and disposition of the roots would bear a relationship to the number and location of the cuspal areas and growth centres within the papilla, thereby establishing a link between the crown pattern and the root pattern.

REFERENCES

Carlson H. (1944) Studies in the role and amount of eruption in certain human teeth. *Am. J. Orthod.* **30,** 575.

Gaunt W. A. (1960) The vascular supply in relation to the formation of roots on the cheek teeth of the mouse. *Acta Anat.* **43,** 116.

Kenney E. B. and Ramfjord S. P. (1969) Cellular dynamics in root forma-tion of teeth in rhesus monkeys. *J. Dent. Res.* **48,** 114.

Lester K. S. (1969) The incorporation of epithelial cells by cementum. *J. Ultrastruct. Res.* **27,** 63.

Noble H. W., Carmichael A. F. and Rankine D. M. (1962) Electron-microscopy of human developing dentine. *Archs Oral Biol.* **7,** 395.

Orban E. and Mueller E. (1929) The development of the bifurcation of multi-rooted teeth. *J. Am. Dent. Ass.* **16,** 297.

Selvig K. A. (1963) Electronmicroscopy of Hertwig's epithelial sheath and of dentine and cementum formation in the mouse incisor. *Acta Odont. Scand.* **21,** 175.

CHAPTER 19

THE PERIODONTIUM

THE periodontium is properly described as the supporting apparatus of the tooth consisting of cement, periodontal ligament, alveolar bone, junctional and sulcular epithelia, the latter being associated with the marginal gingiva. Cement, bone, junctional, and crevicular epithelium are discussed separately and this chapter deals largely with the periodontal ligament. Even so the periodontium should always be considered as the functional unit involved in tooth support.

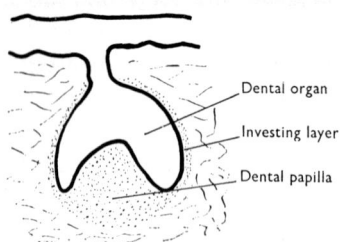

Fig. 82.—Diagram showing the continuity of the dental papilla with the investing layer around the dental organ.

The periodontal ligament is classically described as originating from the dental follicle, that is the mesenchyme between the forming alveolar bone and the developing tooth. However, if the cap and early bell stages of tooth development are examined carefully it can be seen that the ectomesenchyme of the dental papilla continues around the cervical loop of the enamel organ to form an investing layer around the developing tooth (Fig. 82). Recent studies have shown that the cells from this layer give rise to cementoblasts, fibroblasts and osteoblasts which in turn form cement, periodontal ligament and bone. In fact, apart from the gingival component, cells of the investing layer give rise to the entire periodontium. This was established by dissecting out tooth germs at the bell stage of development from day-old mice, labelling the cells of the investing layer with tritiated thymidine and then implanting these tooth germs subcutaneously in adult mice (Fig. 83). In this location the tooth germs continue to develop and three to four weeks later resemble adequately a tooth. Significantly, cement, periodontal ligament, and bone develop in relation to the roots of these subcutaneous teeth.

128

The cementoblasts and ligament fibroblasts are labelled with tritated thymidine, thus establishing their origin from the implanted tooth germ. That the bone cells originated from the same source was established by demonstrating lymphocytes (graft rejection cells) in relation to subcutaneous bone. Interestingly enough in some instances the teeth in this subcutaneous location 'erupted' through the skin with the establishment of an epithelial attachment. These experiments complement previous *in vitro* studies which showed that, when tooth germs were permitted to survive in culture for thirty days, only a few scattered epithelial and ectomesenchymal cells survived. However, when these few cells were harvested and transferred to a connective tissue site, the base of the mouse tail

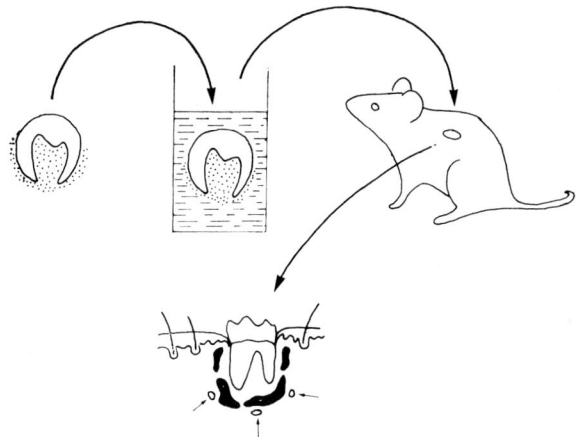

Fig. 83.—Experimental evidence for the origin of the periodontium. A dissected tooth germ is radioactively labelled in a solution of thymidine and implanted beneath the skin of a mouse. The tooth together with periodontal ligament and alveolar bone are all formed. Rejection cells (arrowed) develop on the outer surface of the 'alveolar' bone.

tendon, they resumed their developmental potential and formed a tooth with associated cement, periodontal ligament and bone.

These types of experiments have been extended a little further. If the soft supporting tissues of the tooth are formed from the 'investing layer' it should be possible to implant tooth germs into bone, rather than into soft connective tissue, and form a true gomphosis by fusion of pre-existing bone with the bone generated by the tooth germ. This has been demonstrated to be the case in the following way. When a hole is drilled in the rodent parietal bone, the hole, for some reason, does not fill with bone during repair, but instead becomes filled with fibrous tissue. If a tooth germ is placed into a similar hole the tooth continues development and forms its own supporting tissue, including new bone, which fuses with the old parietal bone. Thus a true gomphosis forms. Whilst an account of these sort of experiments may seem to be rather irrelevant, and a discussion of the origin of the periodontium academic, information of this nature may well be of future significance in relation to tooth germ transplants and the reimplantation of teeth.

It used to be the practice to root-fill and clean the root surface (removing periodontal ligament) of avulsed teeth before reimplanting them back into their sockets. When this was done re-attachment occurred by means of ankylosis; that is fusion of bone with tooth. If attempts are made to preserve adherent periodontal ligament of avulsed teeth before reimplantation the chances of regenerating a normal attachment are increased. Indeed experiments have shown that if avulsed teeth are maintained in a tissue culture medium, permitting growth of adherent periodontal ligament before re-implantation the chances of regenerating an attachment are even better. This is because of the specific embryological origin of the periodontal ligament.

Returning to its histology, the main fibre groups of the periodontal ligament are adequately described in the literature and their anatomy is not considered here. Surprisingly, little is known about the development of the principal fibre groups of the periodontal ligament. It has been suggested that the principal oblique fibres are orientated at the time of root development, an arrangement which is initially seen in histological sections as an oblique orientation of fibroblasts. However, this is not yet certain and it is also claimed that the development of oblique fibre groups does not occur until the tooth bears an axial load after eruption. It is quite possible that species differences exist.

The configuration of the oblique fibres suggests that they function as ties uniting the root to the alveolus; and under load these fibres transmit the force as tension to the alveolar bone. Indeed, the oblique fibres are classically described as having a wavy configuration in the relaxed state but that they straighten out under load. However, there is now a great deal of evidence which shows that this concept is too simplified. For example, if the fibres of the periodontal ligament are cut on the mesial and distal aspects of the tooth, little increase in horizontal mobility occurs, indicating that the fibres are not important in resisting horizontal force. Frequently, when dried skulls are examined, fenestrations in the labial wall of the alveolus not associated with pathological lesions are seen, indicating that a complete bony alveolus is not necessary for tooth support. Under axial load it has been shown that the bony margins of the socket supporting the tooth dilate. If this axial load were converted to tension on the socket wall, as suggested by the orientation of the fibres, the reverse would be anticipated.

This finding can be explained if a compressional system, as well as a tensional system, plays a significant part in tooth support. The ligament can be considered as a compressive hydraulic buffer consisting of a vascular component and a tissue fluid component. The suggestion is that under axial compression, the vascular elements are occluded, followed by the displacement of tissue fluid. However, it has been shown that the periodontal vessels of the monkey incisor unexpectedly failed to collapse when measured pressures were applied to the tooth, and it has been suggested that the maintenance of the patency of blood-vessels under pressure is a function of the oxytalan fibres found in the periodontal ligament. Oxytalan fibres are considered to be a variant of elastic tissue and have been shown to have a distribution within the periodontal ligament closely linked to blood-vessels. Thus they are found to run obliquely between vessels and cement, mainly perpendicular to the occlusal plane and at right angles to the direction of the collagen. The insertion of oxytalan fibres into cement implies an anchorage for the vessels which may permit them to accommodate distortion and compression strains.

The other component of this postulated hydraulic buffer mechanism, the tissue fluid, is considered to be more significant in terms of tooth support. As fluids are incompressible, the cells and extracellular fluid must be displaced if a tooth is pushed into its socket. Where the fluid is displaced is not known, it probably varies with the type of force. If the tooth is subjected to a horizontal force there is some degree of tilt and fluid can be displaced from a region of compression towards a region of tension. Under axial load the fluid can be displaced through the socket wall which is extensively perforated by foramina distributed mainly in the cervical and apical thirds. Also the outward displacement of the socket margin under axial compression suggests tissue fluid displacement towards the rim of the socket. In this case the collagen fibres might act as ties preventing over-dilation of the socket.

When the periodontium is considered it is usually thought of in relation to a single tooth. However, recent studies have indicated further connexions between the periodontium of adjacent teeth in addition to the long established transseptal fibre system. Thus gingival fibres have been described running from one tooth to the adjacent tooth, as have ligament fibres passing through septal bone. It is most likely that some of these fibres are responsible for approximal (mesial or distal) drift, that is movement of the teeth to maintain approximal contact. Thus it has been shown that teeth, isolated from masticatory forces and from the cheeks, tongue and lips, drift continuously and that, if the transseptal group of fibres is severed, a reduction in drift occurs.

A curious feature of the periodontal ligament is the persistence of the fragmented remnants of Hertwig's epithelial root sheath in the form of a network, the epithelial cell rests of Malassez. These persistent epithelial cells in the periodontal ligament serve no known function and indeed are not found in some species. In man the epithelial cell rests have been shown to be viable in the mature ligament and to have the histochemical and ultrastructural features of resting cells. It has been shown *in vitro* and *in vivo* that they retain their ability to divide and migrate under altered environmental conditions and form the epithelial lining of dental cysts.

Another controversial feature of the anatomy of the periodontium is the so-called 'intermediate plexus'. The concept here is that in the middle region of the ligament the collagen of the principal fibre bundles is constantly being broken and reformed to permit tooth movement in an occlusal direction. It has been argued that the histological demonstration of an intermediate plexus in longitudinal sections of teeth *in situ* may be due to the fact that fibres are cut obliquely in the middle of the ligament and radially towards its periphery. No intermediate plexus can be demonstrated in transverse sections through the ligament. However, although the bright field light microscopic appearance of an intermediate plexus may be artefactual, polarized light microscopy indicates that the collagen fibres in the central zone of the ligament are less mature. Also, in experimental avitaminosis C, which interferes with collagen production, the intermediate zone of the ligament shows the greatest degree of disruption which suggests that this is the most active site of collagen synthesis. Radiobiological studies have not helped as much as might have been anticipated. Studies using radioactive proline have not demonstrated remodelling in a clear cut intermediate zone. Instead a fairly even pattern of remodelling occurs with the lowest activity towards the cement surface of the tooth.

However, the above studies indicate that the periodontium has an exceptionally high rate of remodelling and turnover, probably the highest of any connective tissue, and that this involves the degradation and synthesis of collagen. Electron microscopic and histochemical examination of the periodontal ligament has shown that its fibroblasts are capable of phagocytosing and degrading collagen as well as synthesizing this material. Furthermore, these ultrastructural studies provide no evidence for an intermediate plexus. The fact that ligament fibroblasts are able to synthesize and degrade collagen explains how adaptation of ligament might take place during both eruption, function and tooth movement.

The periodontal ligament, in addition to its supportive role, also has an important role as a sensory receptor: a grain of sand in a sandwich is readily detected by receptors in the periodontal ligament. The periodontal ligament contains nerve-fibres running from the apical region towards the gingival margin which are joined by fibres entering the ligament laterally through the foramina of the socket wall. The latter divide into two, with one branch running apically and the other gingivally. The manner in which these nerve fibres terminate has been clarified recently. Some fibres are thought to terminate as free unmyelinated nerve endings and to be associated with pain. Others terminate in specific mechanoreceptors and two types have been described possibly associated with the recognition of elastic deformation and with the recognition of viscous transmission of pressure. It has also been suggested that these structural variations of mechanoreceptors are not really important and that it is their spatial arrangement within the ligament that is the determining factor in their response characteristics. The blood supply of the ligament is dealt with in Chapter 8.

REFERENCES

Anderson A. A. (1967) The protein in matrixes of the teeth and periodontium in hamsters: a tritiated proline study. *J. Dent. Res.* **46**, 67.

Anderson D. J., Hannam A. G. and Mathews G. (1970) Sensory mechanisms in mammalian teeth and their supporting structures. *Physiol. Rev.* **50**, 171.

Birn H. (1966) The vascular supply of the periodontal membrane. *J. Periodont. Res.* **1**, 51.

Carmichael G. C. (1968) Observations with the light microscope on the distribution and connexions of the oxytalan fibre of the lower jaw of the mouse. *Archs Oral Biol.* **13**, 765.

Carneiro J. and Fava de Moraes F. (1965) Radioautographic visualization of collagen metabolism in the periodontal tissues of the mouse. *Archs Oral Biol.* **10**, 833.

Eccles J. D. (1964) The development of the periodontal membrane in the rat incisor. *Archs Oral Biol.* **9**, 127.

Freeman E., Ten Cate A. R. and Dickinson J. (1975) Development of a gomphosis by tooth germ implants in the parietal bone of the mouse. *Archs Oral Biol.* **20**, 139.

Hindle M. O. (1967) The intermediate plexus of the periodontal membrane. In: Anderson D. J., Eastoe J. E., Melcher A. H. and Picton D. C. A. (ed.), *Mechanisms of Tooth Support: A Symposium*. Bristol, Wright, p. 66.

Main J. H. P. (1966) Retention of potential to differentiate in long term culture of tooth germs. *Science, N.Y.* **152**, 778.

Melcher A. H. and Bowen W. H. (1969) *The Biology of the Periodontium*. New York, Academic.

Moss J. P. and Picton D. C. A. (1970) Mesial drift of teeth in adult monkeys (*Macaca irus*) when forces from the cheeks and tongue had been eliminated. *Archs Oral Biol.* **15**, 979.

Muhlemann H. R. and Zander H. A. (1954) Tooth mobility (III). The mechanism of tooth mobility. *J. Periodont.* **25**, 128.

Parfitt G. J. (1967) The Physical Analysis of the Tooth Supporting Structures. In: Anderson D. J., Eastoe J. E., Melcher A. H. and Picton D. C. A. (ed.), *Mechanisms of Tooth Support. A Symposium.* Bristol, Wright, p. 154.

Picton D. C. A. (1965) On the part played by the tooth socket in tooth support. *Archs Oral Biol.* **10**, 945.

Picton D. C. A. (1967) The effect on tooth mobility of trauma to the mesial and distal regions of the periodontal membrane in monkeys. *Helv. Odont. Acta* **11**, 105.

Picton D. C. A. (1969) The effect of external forces on the periodontium. In: Melcher A. H. and Bowen W. H. (ed.), *The Biology of the Periodontium.* New York, Academic, pp. 363–421.

Picton D. C. A. and Moss J. P. (1973) The part played by the transseptal fibre system in experimental approximal drift of the cheek teeth of monkeys (*Macaca irus*). *Archs Oral Biol.* **18**, 669.

Ten Cate A. R. (1969) The development of the periodontium. In: Melcher A. H. and Bowen W. H. (ed.), *Biology of the Periodontium.* New York, Academic, pp. 53–90.

Ten Cate A. R. (1975) Formation of supporting bone in association with periodontal ligament organization in the mouse. *Archs Oral Biol.* **20**, 137.

Ten Cate A. R., Mills C. and Solomon G. (1971) The development of the periodontium. A transplantation and autoradiographic study. *Anat. Rec.* **170**, 365.

Ten Cate A. R. and Mills C. (1972) The development of the periodontium: the origin of alveolar bone. *Anat. Rec.* **173**, 69.

Ten Cate A. R. (1974) The role of the fibroblast in collagen turnover in the functioning periodontal ligament of the mouse. *Archs Oral Biol.* **19**, 339.

Ten Cate A. R., Deporter D. A. and Freeman E. (1976) The role of fibroblasts in the remodelling of periodontal ligament during physiological tooth movement. *Am. J. Orthod.* In the press.

CHAPTER 20

TOOTH ERUPTION

THE forces which move a tooth as it erupts are not yet properly understood. In consequence several theories of tooth eruption exist involving the separate tissues of the dento-alveolar complex. Evidence to support three of these theories consistently appears and it is most likely that the mechanism for eruption can be explained by one or a combination of these three theories. The three theories implicate proliferation of the cells involved in root growth; pressure generated by vascular tissues; and a contractile element within the periodontal ligament.

Most investigations into tooth eruption have made use of the continuously erupting rodent incisor which is permitted to erupt unimpeded by constantly removing the erupted tip of the tooth. Whilst it could be argued that eruption of the very specialized rodent incisor is unlike eruption for other teeth, there are sufficient parallels, not discussed here, to validate the use of this tooth in the study of eruption.

Perhaps the most significant evidence implicating the periodontal ligament comes from a series of simple experiments involving surgical interference with the growing root of the tooth. In one set of experiments (*Fig. 84*) the proliferating enamel organ and dental papilla of the continuously growing lower incisor of the rat were removed. This eliminated any eruptive force which might have been contributed by cellular proliferation in the forming root. After this procedure the tooth continued to erupt at its normal rate until, because there was no formation of new tissues, the tooth was exfoliated. The fact that the only unoperated dental tissue remaining in this experiment was the periodontal ligament suggests that it provided the force for eruption, perhaps by 'pulling' the tooth out of the socket. However, it could be argued that the inflammatory response to surgical interference led to an accumulation of tissue fluid behind the erupting tooth, and that this fluid, under pressure, was responsible for pushing the tooth out of its socket. Against this interpretation it was argued that if tissue fluid pressure had built up behind the erupting tooth it would have pushed fluid out of the exposed pulp canal (the incisal edge of the tooth was continually cut away to allow unimpeded eruption) (*Fig. 84c*). But it is possible that the exposed, empty, pulp chamber was blocked by clotted inflammatory exudate.

To investigate the above problem further, the enamel organ from the labial side of a rodent incisor was removed, thereby preventing any further development of the labial side of the tooth (*Fig. 85*). Ultimately, only the newly developed lingual side of the tooth,

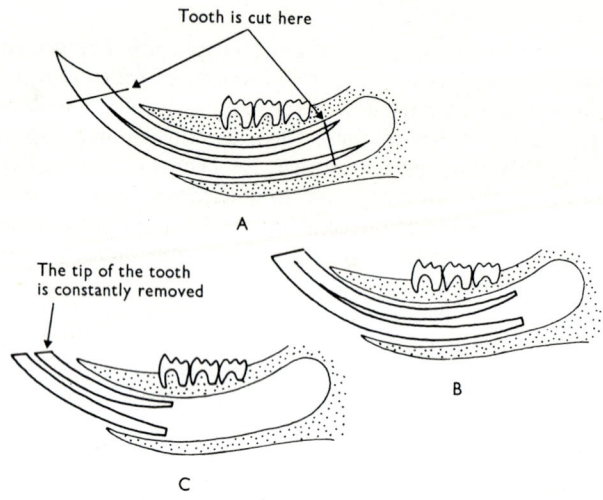

Fig. 84.—The rodent incisor continues to erupt after its forming end has been surgically removed. The incisal edge of the tooth is constantly removed in order to allow it to erupt more rapidly.

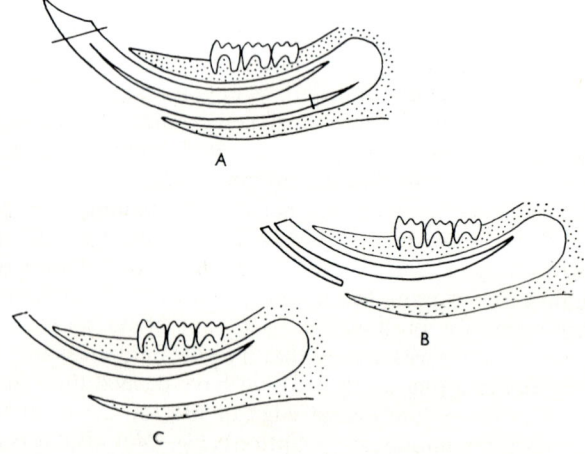

Fig. 85.—The buccal side of the developing end of a rodent incisor is removed. The isolated lingual side continues to develop and erupt.

136

consisting of dentine and cement, remained (*Fig. 85C*); and this continued to erupt. It could be argued either that this fragment was pulled out by the periodontal ligament, or that tissue fluid pressure pushed the fragment out.

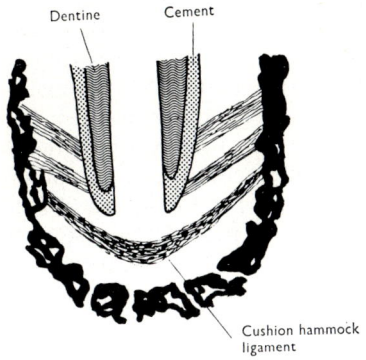

Fig. 86.—Diagram showing the location of the 'cushion hammock ligament'.

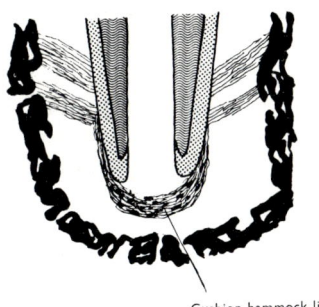

Fig. 87.—Diagram showing the correct interpretation of the so-called 'cushion hammock ligament'.

Some elegant measurements have been made of tissue fluid pressure below and above erupting, but as yet unerupted, teeth in the dog. These have demonstrated that there is a pressure differential of about 15 g, which is more than sufficient to account for eruption.

The above experiments indicate that either contraction of the periodontal ligament or tissue fluid pressure, or both, could provide the force required to pull or push a fragment of tooth out of the jaws.

Turning now to growth of the periapical tissues (proliferating pulp tissues, cement growth or increase in root length), earlier studies seemed to show that tooth eruption was unaffected by drugs which inhibited cell division. Later experiments, in which the dosage of the drugs was increased, showed that tooth eruption was severely retarded. This suggests that cell proliferation is necessary for eruption of the normal tooth. But the experiment does not tell us which are the important cells in this context.

We are still left with three mechanisms which might generate an eruptive force: tissue fluid pressure, cell proliferation and contraction of some element in the periodontal ligament.

Two other theories of eruption should also be briefly mentioned. When the whole of root formation is considered, including epithelial proliferation, dentine deposition and pulpal proliferation, it has been suggested that increase in the length of the forming root provides the eruptive force by pushing against a structure termed the 'cushion hammock ligament'. This structure was described as passing from one side of the socket, under the root apex, to the opposite wall of the socket and its function was thought to be to convert the downward thrust exerted by the growing root into a pull on the socket wall. It has now been clearly demonstrated that this structure is an artefact (*Fig. 86*) and is really a pulp delineating membrane with no connexion to the bone of the socket wall (*Fig. 87*).

Bony remodelling of the jaws has also been linked with tooth eruption. It has been suggested that the inherent growth pattern of the mandible or maxilla moves teeth by selective deposition and resorption of bone in the immediate neighbourhood of the tooth. Elegant and careful studies with tetracyclines as bone markers disprove this theory. Tetracyclines become incorporated in newly formed bone and can be identified in sections due to their fluorescent properties. With the onset of tooth eruption bone is resorbed at the base of the socket. However, this is followed by deposition of bone on the socket floor. Measurements show that the amount of bone deposited, plus the amount of root growth, together equal the distance that the tooth moves, which is scarcely surprising. However, some workers seem to consider that this implicates bone growth with tooth eruption, despite the initial resorption of bone as the tooth begins to move in an occlusal direction. It is more likely that the later deposition of bone is an infilling after the tooth has moved: it is an effect, not a cause, of eruption.

We now return to the three theories mentioned earlier. Theoretically it seems possible that by opening precapillary sphincters at the base of an erupting tooth the tissue fluid pressure in this region could be increased to the extent that sufficient pressure would be generated to push the tooth out of the socket. In a very different situation, everyone is aware of the pressure which can be generated within a boil in the skin before it 'bursts'.

With regard to cell proliferation, it is unfortunate that no single cell population (for example, pulp fibroblasts, root sheath cells, or periodontal fibroblasts) can be destroyed without interfering with other cells. Therefore although cell proliferation appears to be necessary to maintain normal tooth eruption, the force which this activity generates, either directly or indirectly, is not known.

Turning now to the periodontal ligament, either the cells of the ligament or the extracellular collagen are thought to provide the force for tooth movement. Collagen is formed in the ligament. The collagen macromolecules secreted by the fibroblasts are initially arranged in a random fashion in the extracellular compartment. When these macromolecules become ordered to form collagen fibres, there is a decrease in entropy and this decrease in disorder must provide a force along the axis of the orientating fibres to prevent the macromolecules from returning to their disordered state. A reasonable analogy here is a stretched elastic band. When stretched the molecules are in an orderly state (decreased entropy) and there is a contractile force as the molecules try to assume a more disordered state.

Also, as the tropocollagen molecules aggregate to form collagen fibrils by the development of co-valent cross linkage bonds, a contraction of about 10 per cent is thought to occur plus a further contraction due to dehydration. Thus, during collagen fibre formation a tensional force may develop: (1) due to decrease in entropy by electrostatic attraction of disordered collagen molecules; (2) by linear polymerization producing a decrease in length of macromolecules; and (3) by shrinkage due to dehydration. This is one theoretical way the ligament could provide a force. The cells of the forming ligament may also provide a force akin to the contractile force which has been demonstrated in the healing wound. In this situation the cell has been directly implicated, rather than the collagen of the scar.

In the last edition of this book it was suggested that the collagen traction concept was the most plausible source of the eruptive force within the periodontal ligament. This suggestion was based on the results of an experiment using a lathyritic agent to interfere with collagen synthesis. Lathyritic agents exert their effect by disturbing the formation of cross linkages between the macromolecules of tropocollagen. Administration of lathyrogens to experimental animals retards the eruption of teeth (*but see later*). When sections are prepared it is found that the architecture of the forming ligament is disrupted. Significantly, root formation is not affected and the growing root impinges on the floor of the socket with resorption of bone and buckling of the root. Also growth of Hertwig's root sheath is undisturbed and the predentine of the root, the pulpal tissue, and the vascular elements appear normal. Thus the experimental prevention of normal collagen formation in the ligament apparently prevents tooth eruption. It may be asked why it is that in this situation only the collagen of the forming ligament and not the collagen of the forming dentine of the root and alveolar bone is affected. It appears that there is a significant difference between soft tissue collagens and hard tissue collagens and that this difference lies in the nature of the cross linkages between tropocollagen molecules.

However, this experiment has been repeated and expanded with the additional step added of resecting the root. Contrary to the previous study, it was shown that the unimpeded eruption rate in lathyrogenic animals does not differ significantly from control animals. Yet ligament architecture was disrupted. Controls for these experiments were adequate. Until such time as the discrepancy between the above two studies can be explained the view that the eruption is produced by collagen contraction remains unproved.

On the other hand, the suggestion that the ligament fibroblasts may provide a contractile mechanism begins to look more possible. Fibroblasts are contractile cells and it has been reported that when seen in repair tissue, some of their structural features resemble those of smooth muscle cells. These include an extensive filament system, crenulated nuclei and maculae adhaerentes between the cells. Furthermore, fibroblasts in repair tissue have been demonstrated to have similar pharmacological responses to smooth muscle cells. Fibroblasts with similar structural features may be identified in the periodontal ligament. If fibroblasts are responsible for causing the contractions seen in the repair of wounds, a similar contraction might lead to tooth eruption. This possibility should be explored further.

In conclusion, therefore, it seems that the periodontal ligament plays a key role in tooth eruption and it seems likely that the force which is generated has a cellular basis. It is also probable that tissue fluid pressure plays a part at some time in the eruptive cycle—perhaps before the tooth breaks through the oral mucosa.

REFERENCES

Berkovitz B. K. B. (1971) The effect of root transection and partial root resection on the unimpeded eruption rate of the rat incisor. *Archs Oral Biol.* **16**, 1033.

Berkovitz B. K. B. (1971) The healing process in the incisor tooth socket of the rat following root resection and exfoliation. *Archs Oral Biol.* **16**, 1045.

Berkovitz B. K. B. (1972) The effect of preventing eruption on the proliferative basal tissues of the rat lower incisor. *Archs Oral Biol.* **17**, 1279.

Berkovitz B. K. B. (1972) The effect of the lathyritic agent amino-aceto-nitrite on the unimpeded eruption rate in normal and root resected rat lower incisors. *Archs Oral Biol.* **17,** 1755.

Berkovitz B. K. B. and Thomas N. R. (1969) Unimpeded eruption in the root-resected lower incisor of the rat with a preliminary note on root transection. *Archs Oral Biol.* **14,** 771.

Jenkins G. N. (1966) *The Physiology of the Mouth*, 3rd ed. Oxford, Blackwell Scientific.

Main J. H. P. (1965) A histological survey of the hammock ligament. *Archs Oral Biol.* **10,** 343.

Main J. H. P. and Adams D. (1966) Experiments on the rat incisor into the cellular proliferation and blood-pressure theories of tooth eruption. *Archs Oral Biol.* **11,** 163.

Ness A. R. (1964) In: Staple P. H. (ed.), *Advances in Oral Biology*, vol. 1. New York, Academic, pp. 33–70.

Ten Cate A. R. (1969) The mechanism of tooth eruption. In: Melcher A. H. and Bowen W. H. (ed.), *The Biology of the Periodontium*. New York, Academic, pp. 91–103.

Van Hassel H. J. and McMinn R. G. (1972) Pressure differential favouring tooth eruption in the dog. *Archs Oral Biol.* **17,** 183.

CHAPTER 21

THE DENTO-GINGIVAL JUNCTION

ONCE it has erupted, the tooth is surrounded by the only natural break in the living epithelium of the body. Other ectodermal appendages, such as, for example, nails or glands, form invaginations with a complete lining of epithelium. The natural break in epithelial continuity unfortunately represents a weak point and is the site of onset of most periodontal lesions. Because of this the dento-gingival junction has been extensively studied in recent years and our understanding of this region has increased considerably.

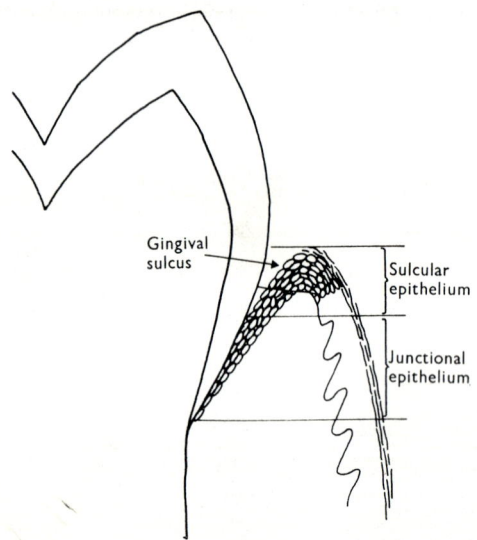

Fig. 88.—Terms used when describing the dento-gingival junction.

Before discussing this region in detail it is necessary to clarify its terminology. Most textbooks use the term 'epithelial attachment' but this properly describes just that part of the dento-gingival complex which actually attaches to dental tissue and provides the biological mechanism which unites epithelial cells to the tooth surface. In this account it is proposed to use the terms outlined in *Fig. 88.* Thus the gingival margin to the bottom of the gingival sulcus is lined by sulcular or crevicular epithelium. The epithelium from the base of the sulcus to its most apical extension is called 'junctional' epithelium. This terminology differs slightly from that proposed in a recent monograph on the 'epithelial attachment'. The difficulty in arriving at a satisfactory terminology is due, in part, to lack of a clear understanding of the development of the 'epithelial attachment' and in part to the failure to recognize that supporting connective tissue plays an important role in controlling the expression of its overlying epithelium. We have therefore eliminated the term 'epithelium' from the title of this chapter. The role of connective tissues in the dento-gingival junction will be discussed later.

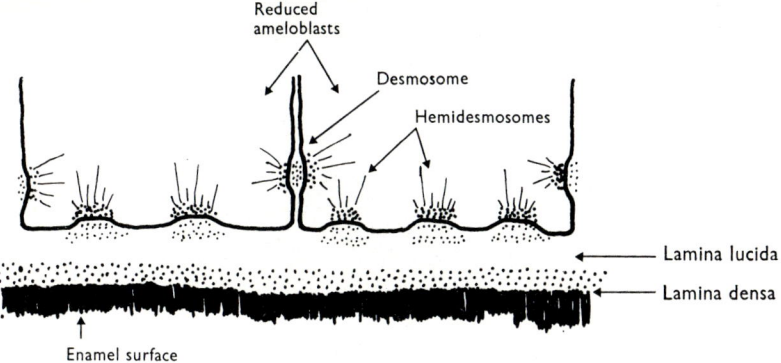

Fig. 89.—Hemidesmosomes in the reduced ameloblasts.

Before doing so the nature of the 'epithelial attachment' can be described because it is now fully understood. Epithelial cells join each other by means of the desmosome. A desmosome consists of components contributed by the two cells in contact with each other (*see Fig. 5c*, p. 10). Where a plasma membrane approaches a region of contact its two layers, as seen with the electron microscope, thicken considerably. The cytoplasm on the inner aspect of this thickened part of the plasma membrane is more electron dense and numerous tonofilaments radiate from here into the cell. This arrangement is repeated in the adjacent cell and a fine electron-dense line can be distinguished in the narrow gap between the two cells (*see* Chapter 2).

Where an epithelial cell is in contact with connective tissue the electron microscope shows that the epithelial cell has hemi-desmosomes (*Fig. 89*), which represent half a desmosome. In addition, two further layers are seen: a lamina lucida and a lamina densa together termed the 'basement lamina'. The mechanism whereby epithelial cells attach to the tooth is identical to the mechanism whereby such cells attach to connective tissue. Thus the epithelial cells adjacent to the enamel surface possess hemi-desmosomes and are in contact with a basement lamina just as in any other epithelial connective tissue junction. The epithelial nature of the attachment can be demonstrated by removing it surgically. Within two months a new attachment forms consisting of hemi-desmosomes and a basement lamina. When the epithelial attachment is to the cement surface instead of enamel (as happens in old age) the attachment is still seen to consist of hemi-desmosomes and a basement lamina.

Thus, the nature of the attachment of the gingiva to tooth is understood. However, it appears that the dento-gingival junction fails to provide an adequate seal to the oral environment and is thus a key factor in the onset of periodontal disease. To understand this problem better an understanding of the development of the dento-gingival junction is necessary.

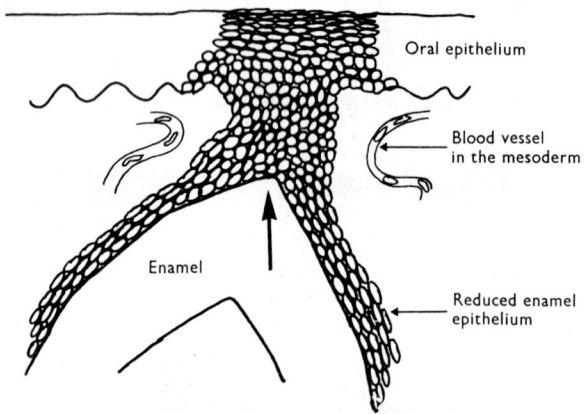

Oral epithelium

Blood vessel
in the mesoderm

Enamel

Reduced enamel
epithelium

Fig. 90.—The tooth erupts through an epithelial plug developed from both oral and dental epithelium.

Before the tooth erupts its enamel surface is covered by the reduced enamel epithelium which consists of an inner layer of reduced ameloblasts and an outer layer of epithelial cells, the remainder of the enamel organ. As the tooth erupts the connective tissue between the reduced enamel epithelium and the oral epithelium is removed and, at the same time, the cells of the outer layer of the reduced enamel epithelium and the basal cells of the oral epithelium prolifer-ate. Thus, a mass of epithelial cells is formed over the tooth and it is through this mass that the tooth erupts, without ever exposing connective tissue to the external environment (*Fig. 90*). This explains why tooth eruption takes place without any haemorrhage.

From this point on there is a degree of uncertainty as to what happens when the dento-gingival junction is established. On the one hand it is possible that basal epithelial cells from the mass over the erupting tooth migrate apically over the remainder of the reduced dental epithelium forming desmosomal attachments with it (*Fig. 91*). On the other hand it is possible that only cells of the reduced dental epithelium become transformed into the junctional epithelium (*Fig. 92*). Whatever the exact occurrence at the time of tooth eruption, it is generally agreed that the reduced enamel epithelium is eventually replaced by the proliferation of other epithelial cells. How this is achieved is not fully understood, but the realization that the epithelial cells are proliferating has transformed the concept of a static junction between gingiva and tooth to one of an actively remodelling junction (*Fig. 93*). No matter what the origin of the epithelial cells constituting the junctional and sulcar epithelium, this epithelium differs significantly from the gingival epithelium in that it is non-keratinized and that its cells are loosely knit instead of tightly packed.

The important controls which determine these differences probably reside in the underlying connective tissue. There are many examples of the dependence of epithelium on its supporting connective tissue and some have already been discussed in Chapter 4 on epithelial mesenchymal relations. Further examples come from simple grafting experiments. If keratinized epithelium *with its supporting connective tissue* is grafted to a non-keratinized site (say to the floor of the vestibular sulcus) the graft remains keratinized. Conversely, if basal epithelial cells from a keratinizing epithelium are seeded onto a bare connective tissue site previously supporting non-keratinized epithelium a non-keratinized epithelium is formed. It is perhaps significant that the connective tissue supporting junctional epithelium is morphologically quite distinct from that supporting gingival epithelium. Thus there are significant differences in the number of collagen fibres present and in the cellular population.

There are very few collagen fibrils, many neutrophils and vesiculated fibroblasts in connective tissue supporting sulcular epithelium whereas the connective tissue supporting gingival epithelium contains many collagen fibres and fibroblasts and no neutrophils or vesiculated fibroblasts. The point has been made that the morphological appearances of the connective tissue supporting sulcular epithelium are similar to, although much less pronounced, than those seen during early gingival inflammation. Thus it would appear that even in clinically healthy gingival tissues some inflammatory changes are present in the connective tissue underlying sulcular epithelium, and it may be that this difference determines the nature of the epithelium in the dento-gingival junction.

For an explanation of why inflammatory changes are present in the supporting connective tissue it is necessary to return again to a consideration of development of the dento-gingival junction. Before doing so, however, it is useful to have some further information concerning epithelial connective tissue relationships. There are now several studies which show that all basal epithelial cells respond in the same way to any disturbance in their supportive connective tissue. These responses include a shift in the basal cells' oxidative cycle from the Krebs cycle to the hexosemonophosphate shunt: lipid synthesis, decreased nuclear cytoplasmic ratio, enlarged extracellular spaces, increased cell division and epithelial migration and, surprisingly, the development of rough endoplasmic reticulum.

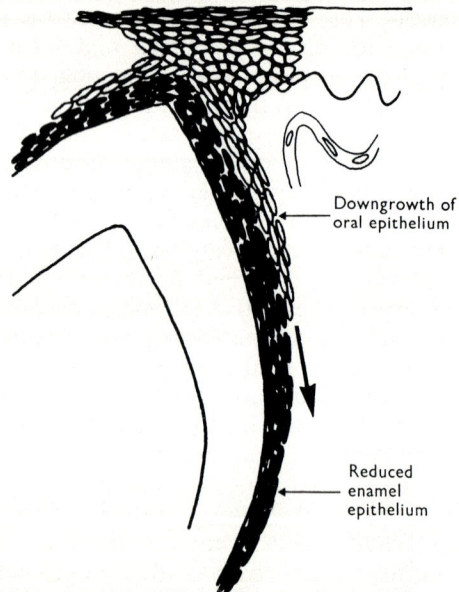

Downgrowth of
oral epithelium

Reduced
enamel
epithelium

Fig. 91.—The development of the dento-gingival junction by migration of cells from the oral epithelium.

If we again consider the situation just before the tooth breaks through the oral epithelium it is apparent that there is connective tissue above and around the crown of the tooth. Both the cells of the reduced dental epithelium and of the oral epithelium respond to the breakdown of this connective tissue by dividing and proliferating through the connective tissues until they fuse. The epithelial cells at this time are separated by widened intercellular spaces and, whilst information is not yet fully available, it is likely that these cells will exhibit the remaining responses already listed for other disturbed epithelia. As soon as the tooth cusp breaks through the oral epithelium, there is a classic inflammatory response from the connective tissue which supports the developing junctional epithelia around the tooth. This implies that antigen has been able to pass through the epithelial complex to stimulate an inflammatory response. The passage of antigen is probably permitted by the wide inter-cellular spaces between the epithelial cells resulting from their response to the physiological breakdown of connective tissue in advance of the erupting tooth. The continued development of junctional epithelium takes place over this connective tissue which is exhibiting acute inflammation.

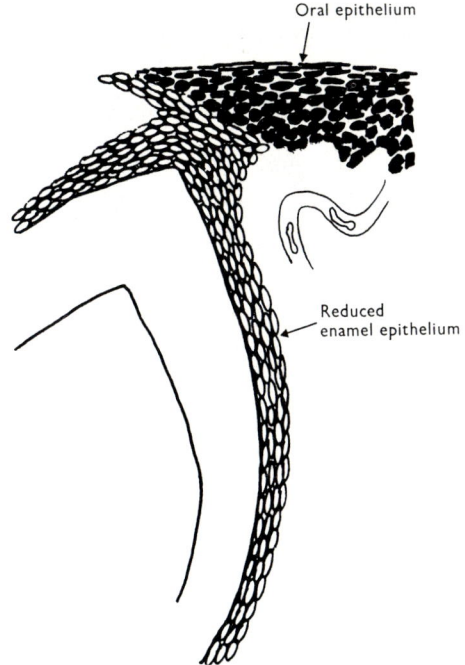

Oral epithelium

Reduced enamel epithelium

Fig. 92.—The development of the dento-gingival junction by trans-formation of dental epithelium.

It is not surprising, therefore, that the junctional epithelium exhibits most of the characteristics of epithelial cells supported by a disturbed connective tissue: namely, wide inter-cellular spaces, high mitotic rate, the presence of rough endoplasmic reticulum and low nuclear cytoplasmic ratio. The acute inflammatory state (clinic-ally seen as 'teething') rapidly subsides after the tooth has broken through the oral epithelium, but with a developing junctional epi-thelium which contains large intercellular spaces, continued ingress

147

of antigens is possible, and could maintain a low grade inflammatory lesion. Hence the explanation for persistent inflammatory change in the supporting connective tissue of sulcular epithelium.

That the spaces between the epithelial cells provide a pathway for antigens has been clearly demonstrated by using labelled bacterial endotoxin as a marker.

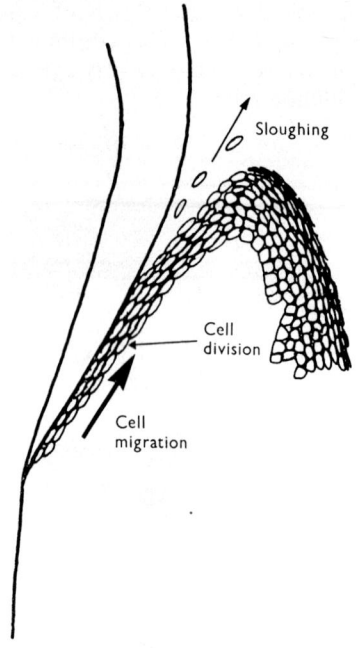

Fig. 93.—Junctional epithelium proliferates and slides up the side of the tooth to be shed into the gingival sulcus.

In conclusion, it is important to think of both the epithelial and connective tissue components in any discussion of the dento-gingival junction. The presence of a disturbed connective tissue supporting junctional epithelium is likely to be due to the persistence of an inflammatory lesion initiated at the time of tooth eruption by the passage of antigens between cells of a developing attachment supported by physiologically disturbed connective tissue resulting from tooth eruption.

REFERENCES

Engler W. O., Ramfjord S. P. and Hiniker J. J. (1965) Development of epithelial attachment and gingival sulcus in Rhesus monkeys. *J. Periodont.* **36**, 44.

148

Glavind L. and Anader H. A. (1970) Dynamics of dental epithelium during tooth eruption. *J. Dent. Res.* **49**, 549.

Listgarten M. A. (1966) Phase contrast and electron microscopic study of the junction between reduced enamel epithelium and enamel in unerupted human teeth. *Archs Oral Biol.* **11**, 999.

Listgarten M. A. (1967) Electron microscopic study of the gingivo-dental junction of man. *Am. J. Anat.* **119**, 147.

Listgarten M. A. (1968) Electron microscopic features of the newly formed epithelial attachment after gingival surgery. A preliminary report. *J. Periodont. Res.* **2**, 46.

Listgarten M. A. (1970) Changing concepts about the dento-epithelial junction. *J. Can. Dent. Ass.* **36**, 70.

Schroeder H. E. and Listgarten M. A. (1971) Fine structure of the developing epithelial attachment in human teeth. In: Wolsky A. (ed.), *Monographs in Developmental Biology*, vol. 2. Basel, Karger.

Stallard R. E., Diab M. A. and Zander H. A. (1965) The attaching substance between enamel and epithelium. A product of the epithelium cells. *J. Periodont.* **36**, 130.

Ten Cate A. R. (1971) Physiological resorption of connective tissue associated with tooth eruption. An electron microscopic study. *J. Periodont. Res.* **6**, 168.

Ten Cate A. R. (1975) The dento-gingival junction. An interpretation of the literature. *J. Periodont.* **46**, 475.

CHAPTER 22

THE FINAL INVESTMENTS OF THE CROWN OF THE TOOTH

AS sometimes happens electron microscopy not only reveals hitherto unobserved structures but also results in interpretations of structures that are quite different from those made by light microscopy. The prism sheaths in enamel were one example of this and the cuticles of the tooth are another.

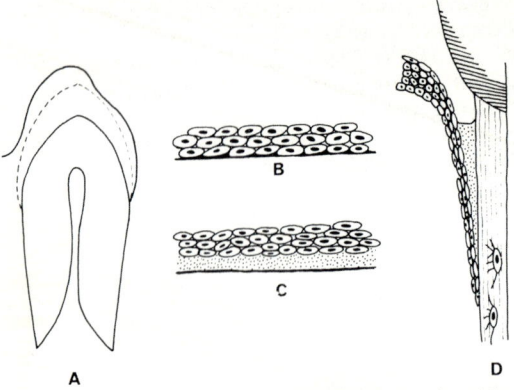

Fig. 94.—When a recently erupted tooth is dissolved in acid a membrane floats from the surface of the dissolved enamel (Nasmyth's membrane, A). This consists of the reduced enamel epithelium and possibly a thin inner structureless layer, the primary enamel cuticle (B). Sometimes a much thicker structureless layer, with different staining properties, intervenes between the two layers (secondary enamel cuticle, stippled in C), although the primary cuticle indicated in this diagram is usually not seen. A secondary enamel cuticle (stippled in D) may also separate the cement from the epithelial attachment.

In the last century the two-layered appearance of a membrane which covers newly erupted teeth was described (*Fig. 94A* and *B*). The outer layer of this membrane is cellular and probably consists entirely of the remnants of the enamel organ which covered the fully developed enamel. For obvious reasons this cellular layer is called the 'reduced enamel epithelium'. The inner layer, about whose presence there has been disagreement, is about 1 μm thick, is not always seen, and has a structureless refractile appearance. It is called the 'primary enamel cuticle' and is perhaps the partially mineralized or unmineralized last formed product of the amelo-blasts. The two layers, cellular and acellular, are known together as 'Nasmyth's membrane'.

A considerably thicker cuticle with different staining properties *may* be seen on the root of the tooth (*Fig. 94D*) and sometimes on the crown of the tooth between the primary cuticle and the reduced enamel epithelium (*Fig. 94C*). This 'secondary' enamel cuticle, which appears to have affinities with the protein of red blood cells, may have a pathological origin.

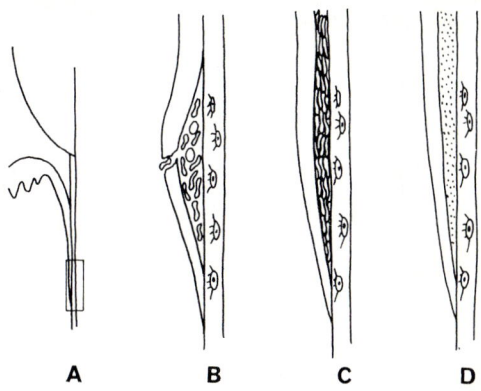

| A | B | C | D |

Fig. 95.—Possible mode of formation of the secondary enamel cuticle in the root region of a tooth. Boxed region in A is shown in B, C, and D.

Blood cells from small haemorrhages in the tooth follicle or periodontal ligament may leak through the epithelial layers lifting either the reduced enamel epithelium or the junctional epithelium away from the surface of the tooth (*Fig. 95B*). The blood cells autolyse and iron becomes absorbed back through the epithelial layers (*Fig. 95C*). The larger molecular weight proteins break down but are not absorbed and remain, what is in effect, outside the body (outside the epithelia). Here they condense together becoming the secondary enamel cuticle (*Fig. 95D*). Particularly convincing has been the demonstration that a layer of red blood cells squashed on to a wax surface can produce *in vitro* a structure which resembles in all ways a secondary enamel cuticle.

However, the above description is altogether too simplified. The reduced enamel epithelium contains two cell types. An inner layer of 'reduced ameloblasts' can be recognized until about the time at which the tooth erupts (*Fig. 96 A–C*). Between the end of amelo-genesis and the eruption of the tooth (a period of about three years for the first permanent molar) these cells 'degenerate' from columnar, to cuboidal, to squamous. They adhere to the surface of the enamel by means of a basement lamina and hemidesmosomes (*Fig. 96 D–E*). The remainder of the cells of the enamel organ (stratum intermedium, external enamel epithelium, and perhaps some stellate reticulum) which, it will be recalled, are already squamous at the end of amelogenesis, become the outer layer of reduced enamel epithelium and are capable of dividing. It is not known what happens in the next year or two but by the time the tooth begins to move towards the oral cavity the enamel is covered by an actively proliferating reduced enamel epithelium which has generated a basement lamina together with the associated hemidesmosomes (Chapter 21).

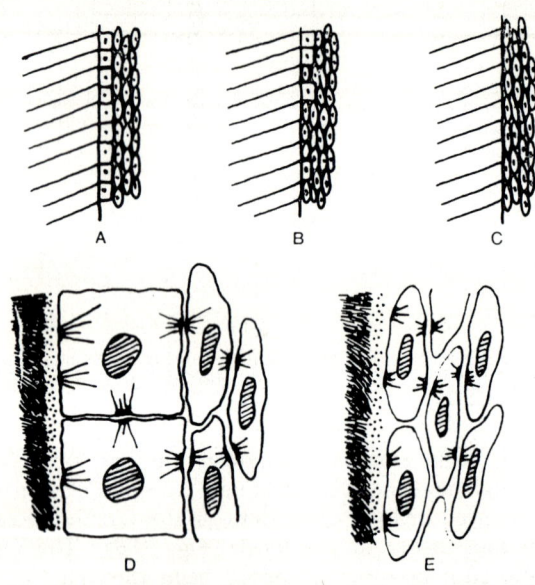

Fig. 96.—The replacement (or conversion) of reduced ameloblasts by more squamous cells (A–C). D and E are high-power views of A and C.

As the tooth erupts, proliferating cells of the reduced enamel epithelium mingle with proliferating cells of the oral epithelium to become what is known as 'junctional epithelium'; i.e. that epithelium which forms a junction between enamel and what is obviously oral epithelium (*Fig. 88*). However, that part of the tooth beyond the junctional epithelium, and well into the oral cavity, may still retain a few adherent cells (? reduced ameloblasts, or cells from the proliferating layer of the reduced enamel epithelium, or perhaps cells from junctional epithelium) (*Fig. 97B*).

152

Several types of cuticle have been described. We have already mentioned the primary enamel cuticle, suggesting that it could be the outer layer of unmineralized enamel matrix. However, it could be a product of the *'reduced* ameloblasts' or of the outer layers of the reduced enamel epithelium, in which case it is most unlikely to have any affinity with the enamel proteins. It is more probable that it would have affinities with basement lamina protein which, it will be recalled, is 'secreted' onto the surface of the enamel when it mediates the attachment of the reduced enamel epithelium. But the thickness of this cuticle (which may be called 'cuticle B' or the 'dental cuticle') is far greater than that of a basement lamina, suggesting that there has been an over-production of basement lamina protein (*Fig. 97B*).

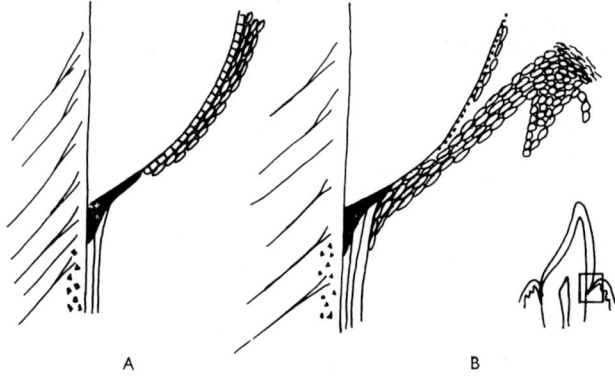

A   B

Fig. 97.—(A) Following crown formation and prior to tooth eruption, the reduced enamel epithelium 'contracts' away from the cervical margin of the tooth exposing enamel to the tooth follicle. Neck cement (black) is laid down. Later, acellular cement is deposited on the neck cement. (B) The cervical enamel of an erupted tooth may be covered by a cuticle of greatly thickened basement lamina material (dotted line). Some cells from the junctional epithelium may adhere to this cuticle.

Unlike the above cuticles, other 'cuticular' structures are mineralized. We have already mentioned that the reduced ameloblasts may degenerate before the tooth has erupted. But, in many animals almost the whole of the enamel epithelium degenerates so that the mesoderm of the tooth follicle comes into contact with the naked enamel. Cementoblasts are differentiated and cement is laid down on the surface of the tooth. Isolated patches of cement have been described on the surfaces of human teeth. However, more commonly the degeneration of enamel epithelium takes place at the neck of the tooth, and in this region a granular, layered structure is laid down (*Fig. 97A*). Because it does not contain collagen fibres it can

153

be distinguished from acellular cement. It has been called 'cuticle A': we suggest that 'neck cement' might be a suitable term.

Other integuments found on the surfaces of teeth are food debris, dental plaque which consists of a soft mass of bacteria, and cellular debris which accumulates rapidly in the absence of oral hygiene, and finally calcified deposits on the tooth surface (calculus). Collectively they can be called 'acquired pellicles'.

Acquired pellicles do not really concern us here. They are, however, of great importance in the onset both of carious lesion and of periodontal disease.

REFERENCES

Dawes C., Jenkins G. N. and Tonge C. H. (1963) The nomenclature of the integuments of the enamel surface of teeth. *Br. Dent. J.* **115,** 65.

Hodson J. J. (1966a) The distribution, structure, origin and nature of the dental cuticle of Gottlieb, Part I and Part II. *J. Am. Soc. Periodont.* **5,** 237, 295.

Hodson J. J. (1966) Electron microscopic study of the gingivo-dental junction of man. *Am. J. Anat.* **119,** 147.

Melcher A. H. and Zarb G. A., ed. (1972) Gingival Epithelium. *Oral Sciences Reviews*, 1. Copenhagen, Munskgaard.

Provenza D. V. and Sisca R. F. (1970) Fine structure features of monkey (*Macaca mulatta*) reduced enamel epithelium. *J. Periodont.* **4,** 313.

For further references, *see* Chapter 21.

CHAPTER 23

AGE CHANGES IN THE DENTAL TISSUES

IN animal wildlife teeth are such important structures that the loss of the dentition marks the end of an animal's life-span. Although this is not true of modern man the teeth exhibit senescent phenomena which are important. Perhaps the most important age changes are the wear of enamel (because it cannot be replaced) and the apical retreat of the epithelial attachment (which must eventually lead to the loss of the tooth).

Enamel is a relatively inert tissue because it has no cellular component. However, certain age changes take place in response to attrition and to physico-chemical changes in structure.

The most conspicuous age change associated with enamel is its loss due to wear. This loss is extremely variable depending on the diet of the individual, the nature of the occlusion, and the composition of the enamel. Attrition of the occlusal surfaces of teeth is obvious. Attrition also occurs at the contact points between teeth due to the differential movements of adjacent teeth during mastication, and the extent of this wear can be considerable. It has been estimated that by the age of 40 as much as 1 cm can be lost from the overall circumferential length of the arch in the average complete dentition.

The use of dyes and radioactive isotopes has shown conclusively that enamel is slightly permeable, and that this permeability decreases with age. It seems that ions are exchanged between the surface enamel and saliva. It is well known that fluorine is most beneficial if the ion is incorporated within the enamel during its development, or absorbed onto its surface immediately after its appearance in the oral cavity. The reduction of the incidence of caries in young individuals exposed to fluoride can be explained by the higher permeability of younger enamel to ions. There is little evidence for any change in the organic content of the enamel with age and this is not surprising in view of the nature of this non-vital tissue. Thus, it can be stated that the changes that are brought about in enamel with increasing age are those of a physico-chemical nature, and result from the interaction between the oral environment and the enamel surface.

Age changes in the dentine are more marked because, unlike enamel, this tissue is vital. The formation of dentine continues throughout life but at a diminishing rate, so that the volume of the pulp chamber progressively diminishes. Recent studies have shown a marked difference in the composition of the matrix of the rapidly formed primary dentine compared with the slowly formed physiological (or regular) secondary dentine. In addition to the deposition of this secondary dentine, dentine is also deposited in response to advancing attrition and dental disease. In response to these stimuli pathological (or irregular) secondary dentine, in which a reduced number of tubules pursue a haphazard course, is deposited. Physiological secondary dentine would appear to be a natural consequence of ageing unrelated to injury of the tooth.

Another age change in dentine, not necessarily related to the pathology of the tooth, is the formation of translucent or sclerotic dentine. Here the tubules of the dentine are progressively occluded, by deposition within their lumens of mineral salts, so that the now mineralized tubules have the same refractive index as inter-tubular dentine. It is thought that the tubules become filled with peri-tubular dentine. Although translucent dentine can develop anywhere in the dentine, it is consistently found in the root region after middle age. Teeth containing translucent dentine appear to be more brittle than other teeth making them more liable to fracture during extraction.

Dead tracts are also found in dentine. Here the odontoblast process degenerates leaving an empty tubule. Such tubules are, however, sealed off at their pulpal end by the deposition of pathological (irregular) secondary dentine. When viewed in transmitted light dead tracts appear more opaque than normal dentine due to the presence of air in the empty tubules. Although translucent dentine and dead tracts frequently form in response to attrition or dental disease, there is ample evidence that both changes can be independent of peripheral injuries, and they must consequently be regarded as progressive age changes within dentine.

Cement is deposited intermittently throughout life around the roots of teeth and there is a loose correlation between the thickness of cement and age. This relationship is a linear one, but the thickness of cement is too readily influenced by the functional stresses applied to the tooth and by periodontal disease, to provide a wholly reliable indication of dental age.

With the initial completion of the apex of the root the dental pulp can be considered to have attained maturity. The pulp has been shown to be similar in comparison, organization, and histochemical reactivity to other connective tissues, and it bears the same relationship to dentine as bone-marrow to mineralized bone. Functionally, pulp and dentine should be regarded as the two parts of one tissue and in consequence some of the age changes of dentine are also age changes of the pulp.

The young pulp contains many fibroblasts, young collagen fibres, and relatively few mature collagen fibres, all disposed in a fluid ground substance. With advancing age, mature collagen fibres increase in number, cellular elements decrease, and the ground substance becomes less aqueous. These changes may be the result of a diminishing blood-supply to the pulp consequent upon vascular strangulation by narrowing of the apical canal and upon progressive arteriosclerosis. It is also claimed that the nerve-supply to the pulp diminishes with increasing age.

Radiographs often reveal the presence of mineralized nodules within the pulp cavity of the tooth. Under the light microscope these 'pulp stones' can have one of two appearances. Either the irregularly mineralized nodules may contain a few randomly arranged tubules or they may have the appearance of a relatively acellular bone. The first type is called a true pulp stone (because it contains 'dentinal tubules'), the second a false pulp stone. With the progressive deposition of dentine on the walls of the pulp cavity these stones may finally become embedded on the encroaching pulpal surface of the dentine. Another variety of ectopic mineralization is referred to as 'diffuse calcification of the pulp'. In this case irregular strands (rather than discrete nodules) of poorly mineralized tissue are found distributed throughout the pulp. The origin of pulp stones is unknown. Perhaps, following a minute pulpal haemorrhage, extravasated blood-cells form a focus for the development of fibrous tissue which subsequently becomes mineralized. Layers of mineralized tissue are now deposited around this focus to form the discrete mineralized nodule. But this cannot explain the presence of 'dentinal tubules' in a pulp stone. It will be recalled that odontoblasts are only differentiated under the influence of the internal enamel epithelium or Hertwig's root sheath and neither of these is present in the pulp. Diffuse calcification of the pulp is probably produced in response to the decreased vascularity of an ageing pulp but the mechanism by which it is produced is not known.

The periodontal ligament forms the attachment between tooth and bone and the life span of the tooth depends upon its integrity. Little is known of the quantitative and qualitative changes occurring with age within the ligament itself except that it may become narrower with age; far more attention has been paid to the apical downgrowth of the epithelial attachment with age. Two opinions have been expressed in attempts to explain the cause of the retreat of the attachment. Some consider it is a direct response to inflammatory change in the periodontal ligament, and it is true that in sections of this region some evidence of inflammatory cell infiltration can always be found. An alternative interpretation is that the retreat of the attachment is a physiological process termed 'passive eruption'. In other animals, where gingival disease is not as widespread as in man, slow gingival recession proceeds as an apparently normal age change and this fact has been used as an argument against the belief that inflammatory change is the causative factor.

Whatever the reason for the retreat of the attachment, it will be appreciated that it must be preceded by the removal of the adjacent gingival fibres of the periodontal ligament and be followed by resorption of the bony alveolar crests. Finally, even if it is accepted that regression is related to age, this does not necessarily mean that this is a physiological ageing process. Taking all the evidence into account, it is most likely that it is the environment of the attachment which results in its downward retreat with age.

Clinical observations give the impression that the oral mucosa in the aged is thinner, dryer and more fragile. However, little work has been done on this problem; such work is urgently required because of its clinical significance. What evidence there is suggests that there is diminution in keratinization with age, but this has been obtained from studies involving cytological smears which at best are capricious.

Studies of teeth have proved exceptionally useful in determining the age of mutilated or otherwise unrecognizable bodies. It is obvious that up to the age of twenty the developing and erupting teeth provide an accurate estimate of an individual's age. However, even beyond this time teeth frequently provide very good estimates of age. Longitudinal ground sections of a single tooth or several teeth are prepared. The following five features are studied: attrition, secondary dentine, translucent dentine, the position of the epithelial attachment and the thickness of the cement. Each of these features is given a score from 0 to 3. Zero represents the condition expected in a perfect young tooth whereas 3 represents an extremely advanced stage of, for instance, spread of translucent dentine, attrition, or cement thickness. The five scores are added together to give a final figure. Thus a single tooth may score attrition 2, secondary dentine 1, translucent dentine 3, epithelial attachment 1, cement 2. The total is 9. By referring to published tables a good estimate of the age of a person having teeth with a score of 9 can be obtained.

REFERENCES

Bernick S. (1967) Age changes in the blood supply to human teeth. *J. Dent. Res.* **46**, 544.

Black G. V. (1924) In: *Operative Dentistry*, 6th ed., vol. 1. London, Kimpton, p. 223.

Gustafson G. (1950) Age determinations of teeth. *J. Am. Dent. Ass.* **41**, 45.

Jenkins G. N. (1966) *The Physiology of the Mouth*, 3rd ed., Oxford, Black-well, pp. 157, 241.

Miles A. E. W. (1961) Ageing in teeth and oral tissues. In: Bourne G. H. (ed.), *Structural Aspects of Ageing*. London, Pitman.

Miles A. E. W. (1963) The dentition in the Assessment of individual age in skeletal material. In: Brothwell D. R. (ed.), *Dental Anthropology*. Oxford, Pergamon.

Phillipas G. G. and Applebaum E. (1966) Age factor in secondary dentine formation. *J. Dent. Res.* **45,** 778.

Zander H. A. and Hürzeleger B. (1958) Continuous cementum apposition. *J. Dent. Res.* **37,** 1035.

159

INDEX

164

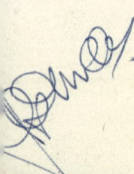